How to do
your Research
Project

This book is dedicated to my parents, John and Pat Beardsmore. They taught me all the important lessons of life.

This title is also available as an e-book.
For more details, please see
www.wiley.com/buy/9780470658208
or scan this QR code:

How to do your Research Project

A guide for students in medicine and the health sciences

Caroline Beardsmore

Senior Lecturer and Postgraduate Tutor
Department of Infection, Immunity and Inflammation (Child Health)
University of Leicester
Leicester Royal Infirmary
Leicester, UK

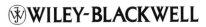

WILEY-BLACKWELL

A John Wiley & Sons, Ltd., Publication

Registered office: John Wiley & Sons, Ltd, The Atrium, Southern Gate, Chichester, West Sussex, PO19 8SQ, UK

Editorial offices: 9600 Garsington Road, Oxford, OX4 2DQ, UK
The Atrium, Southern Gate, Chichester, West Sussex, PO19 8SQ, UK
111 River Street, Hoboken, NJ 07030-5774, USA

For details of our global editorial offices, for customer services and for information about how to apply for permission to reuse the copyright material in this book please see our website at www.wiley.com/wiley-blackwell.

Library of Congress Cataloging-in-Publication Data

Beardsmore, Caroline.
  How to do your research project : a guide for students in medicine and the health sciences / Caroline Beardsmore.
      p. ; cm.
  Includes bibliographical references and index.
  ISBN 978-0-470-65820-8 (softback : alk. paper) – ISBN 978-1-118-64198-9 (eMobi) – ISBN 978-1-118-64225-2 (ePub) – ISBN 978-1-118-64251-1 (ePDF)
    I. Title.
  [DNLM: 1. Biomedical Research.   2. Research Design.   3. Students, Health Occupations.   W 20.5]
    R853.C55
    610.72′4–dc23

                                                                                            2013003016

A catalogue record for this book is available from the British Library.

Cover design by Andy Meaden

Set in 9.5/12pt Minion by Aptara® Inc., New Delhi, India
Printed and bound in Malaysia by Vivar Printing Sdn Bhd

1   2013

Contents

Preface

Many students in medicine and health sciences have an opportunity to carry out a research project. This is a new experience for the majority of students, at once both challenging and daunting. No two projects will be the same, so each student will have to forge their own path. This book is written to help guide you through the whole process from start to finish, in as smooth a way as possible. It can be read in its entirety before embarking on a project, and various chapters re-read at appropriate points during your research.

The book begins with a chapter on how to decide whether or not to take a research option, and what sort of project is most suited to your aims and personality. The book acknowledges that a research project is a requirement of their course for some students, and some have no choice in their project. Projects may be carried out over different lengths of time, and may be analytical (or library) projects, or have a major laboratory or clinical component. Whatever the style of project, the subsequent chapters will show you how to get started, maintain the momentum, achieve the all-important write-up, and prepare for the assessment. A separate chapter is devoted to the supervisor and other colleagues, as research is almost never an individual enterprise and good working relationships are vital. Another chapter discusses how to maximise impact, showing how you can make your own opportunities to promote the results of your research. The final chapter deals with problems you might encounter, so that you can anticipate and avoid them where possible and make modifications to your project if needs be.

Each chapter in the book contains text boxes and examples to illustrate the various points and encourage the reader to think through the relevance for their own project. Several of these examples of students and their projects appear in different chapters to provide some continuity of approach. The majority of examples are based on real situations that have been faced by students and their supervisors. The boxed examples can be used as stand-alone cases for the reader to reflect on, and illustrate the need to think creatively when approaching research.

This book has grown out of my involvement with several cohorts of medical students undertaking an intercalated BSc, in which a research project has been a major (and sometimes the only) component. Although it has been developed primarily for intercalating BSc students, the information and advice it contains is equally applicable to students working in other health-related disciplines. The opportunity to do a research project brings with it many benefits, personal as well as educational, and I hope that this manual will help you, the reader, to gain as much as possible from the experience. My thanks go to all the students and their supervisors who have shared their experiences with me, without which the book would not have been written.

Caroline Beardsmore

Chapter 1 **Before you start**

CHAPTER OVERVIEW

This chapter highlights some of the things to take into account when the student has a choice over whether to take a research project or not. It then covers how to select a project based on the potential supervisor and the student's own skills and abilities. There are suggestions about what to do in advance of starting the project.

Introduction

Doing a piece of research is an opportunity to flex your intellect and showcase your talents in a manner that is not always possible in other parts of a medical or healthcare curriculum. Much is made of integrating knowledge in other parts of your course, but in a research project you will have to integrate knowledge with different skills and abilities that may not have been assessed previously. These may include seeking out and reviewing original research papers, designing your own experimental work, solving problems as they arise, managing your time (and your supervisor!), finding new ways of analysing and presenting data, and writing an extensive report. Research is always a challenge, but one that can be immensely fulfilling for those who engage fully with the process. The rewards of a research project are not limited to any grade or mark you may be assigned at the end, but extend into the less tangible but more long-lasting areas of personal development, independence and a taste for research that may last a lifetime. As with most challenges, preparation is the key. The aim of this manual is to help you rise to the challenge and excel.

How to do your Research Project: A Guide for Students in Medicine and the Health Sciences, First Edition. Caroline Beardsmore.
© 2013 John Wiley & Sons, Ltd. Published 2013 by John Wiley & Sons, Ltd.

What constitutes a research project?

One dictionary definition of 'research' is that it is '. . . systematic investigation towards increasing the sum of knowledge' (Chambers Concise Dictionary, 1991). Within the context of medicine and healthcare, research may evoke images of white-coated scientists working at a laboratory bench, or of doctors administering a new medication to a sick patient. While this may constitute the popular understanding of research, it can encompass other things, including explorations of human attitudes, understanding and behaviour. This illustrates two divisions of research that are commonly recognised: quantitative and qualitative. Quantitative research usually involves something that can be measured (e.g. change in heart rate in response to exercise, proportions of adults in different age categories taking prescribed medications, impact of an added nutrient on growth of cells in culture). The outputs of quantitative research are usually numerical and frequently subjected to statistical analysis. Qualitative research, in contrast, often aims to describe or explain something, and the data are more likely to comprise words than numbers. The outputs may include notes, transcripts or other written records. Qualitative research has its roots in the social sciences and complements quantitative research in many healthcare settings. Discoveries from one type of research may prompt studies in the other; for example, a qualitative study might show that teenage girls are ignorant of the potential health risks of a tattoo, which might then be usefully followed up by a quantitative investigation into the frequency of skin infections and allergic reactions in people going to a tattoo studio. Similarly, a finding that vaccination rates in infants had fallen in a particular area (quantitative research) might prompt a qualitative investigation aiming to explain this. Both types of research are equally valid, although individuals might find they are better suited to one or the other type.

The research projects available for students will vary according to what their educational institution offers. For some, they may have the chance to spend a whole academic year on a research project, whereas others may be of shorter duration and are expected to be done in parallel with other modules or course work. Some students will have the opportunity to learn advanced laboratory techniques that may require considerable practice before meaningful data can be acquired; for others, the time available for the project may mean this is not a possibility. Not all institutions will offer qualitative research. Depending on the institution, projects may not necessarily involve acquiring new data but instead consist of combining data from existing sources and synthesising new information. Such projects are sometimes described as 'analytical' or 'library' projects. While they may not provide the full range of opportunities for maximising impact (see Chapter 6), they still demand the same skills of acquiring information and presenting work as any other research project.

Should I take the research project option or not?

A research project is a requirement for some students and an option for others. Whether it is a requirement or not, it is worthwhile spending some time considering why you might be doing research and what you can do beforehand to ensure that you get the best experience and outcome possible. For some, the initial decision will be whether to take a research option or not. The next step, assuming that you have a choice in the matter, is to think about what sort of project you would like to do and what will best fit with your personal strengths. Where possible, you should explore your options concerning your project and the implications for your career and personal development well in advance of starting.

If your research is optional and involves an extension to your course then you may have several things to consider.

Financial implications

An extra year, as a student, will involve some expense, unless you are fortunate enough to have a full scholarship or bursary and is likely to postpone your opportunity to earn a professional salary for a year. Can you afford to do this? The extra year, however, might well give you an advantage over other applicants when you come to apply for a job so that if you want to work in a very competitive specialty, the research could be a big advantage. The personal and financial circumstances of every student are different and only you can decide if any financial sacrifice is possible or worthwhile. If you have an opportunity to carry out a research project that does not require a full year, such as something extending over the summer vacation, then the financial aspects are less significant.

Timing

The timing of an extra year can be significant. This may be outside your control but not necessarily so. If you take the extra year late in your course (e.g. between years 4 and 5 of medical school) you can find that you are facing your final examinations soon after returning to the main curriculum, and you may not have had much time to revise and practise your clinical skills. Organising some extra sessions for yourself may pay dividends.

Taking an extra year will mean that you fall behind your peer group and will graduate later than they do. This may be offset by having friends who are likely to want to take the extra year, but in any case you will quickly settle into another cohort of students when you return to the main curriculum.

Motivation

Consider carefully your motivation for wanting to do a research project. Many students see it as advantageous to their career, and few would disagree with this. There is nothing wrong with wanting to advance your career; many people do this throughout their working lives and in many ways. If your sole motivation is career advancement, however, you will find your research project very tough going and you might be better advised to look for other routes. If you want the opportunity to try your hand at research, with a possible view to having a research element in your future career, then an early chance to experience research at first hand is invaluable. If there is something that has sparked your professional interest during the early stages of your course then you may be able to explore this in your research project.

Some students, particularly medical students with a very full curriculum, like the idea of 'stepping off the treadmill' of relentless lectures, tutorials, clinical sessions, ward rounds, frequent assessments and so on for a year to do something very different. A research project will certainly enable you to do this. Do not, however, regard it as a 'soft option'. Almost without exception, project students will report afterwards that they never realised how hard they would have to work. You may be considering taking an additional role or commitment (e.g. being an officer in the student's union, or being your university's representative on a national student organisation, or participating at a national level in a particular sport that requires a heavy commitment to training) and you might think that a year, as a project student, will allow you to do this. This may indeed be the case, as you could find yourself with a more flexible schedule than you have previously experienced, but do not imagine that you can complete a good research project without putting in the necessary time, effort and energy.

Occasionally, a student will be considering whether their original choice of course or career was the correct one for them. Under these circumstances, an extra year (or a period of several months) will provide an opportunity to reflect on matters. If it becomes clear that a change of career is in the student's best interest, then he or she will have additional experience and possible qualifications to help them move to the next stage of their professional journey.

Involving others in your decision

Students sometimes agonise over the decision about whether to take a research project option. If you are in this category, draw a line down a piece of paper and write two lists – the advantages and disadvantages of doing a research project. Be completely honest: the list is for your eyes only unless you decide to share it. Then think about any other people who might be directly affected by your decision. Students planning to marry often wait until after graduation; how will your fiancé(e) feel if you extend your course? If someone else is providing financial support, are they able (and willing) to cover the additional costs? Talk about the advantages and disadvantages with others who will be affected by your decision.

Whether or not there are other people likely to be affected by your decision, or those who are affected support you (whatever decision you make), you would be well advised to talk to a range of other people to ascertain their views. These are likely to include your personal tutor, professionals at different stages of their career and senior students. Find out why they did (or did not) take the opportunity to do a research project themselves, and what they perceive as the strengths and weaknesses of taking the extra time. You are likely to find a range of opinions, but what you must think about is the reasons behind the different views and how these relate to your own thinking and circumstances. For example, a senior clinician may say 'the research experience may be valuable, but when I am short-listing candidates for a job I pay more attention to the extent of clinical experience'. Such a comment would have more impact on a student whose motivation is geared towards career advancement than on a student who is driven to explore a particular topic in more depth. Ultimately, the decision may be yours alone but is likely to be even more difficult if you cannot be assured of your research topic or supervisor.

What if your institution is selective?
If your institution selects or invites certain students to undertake a research project, and you have received the flattering e-mail or letter asking you to consider this option, then obviously those who oversee your academic performance consider that it would be in your interests to do so. Go and talk to the course convener or other responsible person to ask about the various options that might be open to you. If you are concerned about the financial implications, be completely open about this. You may find that there are bursaries available, or you could be put forward for an award or scholarship. Do not be embarrassed to ask about funding or financial costs for the individual.

If your institution selects students to consider a research project but you have not been included among them, you may want to ask if the opportunity could be extended to you. If the research project is something you feel you really want to do, speak to the people responsible for the scheme at your institution and ask if you could be included. Be prepared for the answer to be 'No', but you might be lucky! If the guidelines are being strictly followed and you are not given the opportunity for a formal research project, then you might consider whether you could offer to assist in some ongoing research, perhaps over a summer vacation, in order to gain some research experience.

How should I choose what I do for my project?

Some institutions may not give you a choice of project, and others may allow you to express a preference but on the understanding that you may not be allocated your first choice. In other places you might find that you can play a part in designing the project from scratch. If you have a choice you will want to spend some time considering it.

When students who have completed their projects have been asked what advice or recommendations they would give to a student considering an intercalated BSc year, the most important factor has been that of choosing the supervisor carefully! The choice of an interesting topic for the research project was considered to be of secondary importance. Topics that initially seemed unappealing often became much more interesting when the students started to get involved in the work. Now it is rather tricky to suggest that students should evaluate the supervisory styles and personalities of their academic staff, but – in essence – this is what you need to do.

How should I choose a supervisor?

Chapter 3 discusses different working relationships, but at this stage you need to find out about the type of supervision you might expect. The potential supervisor may be somebody you already know as a lecturer or tutor, in which case you might have a view about how easy it would be to work under his or her direction. Do not assume that someone who gives excellent lectures would also be a great supervisor, because the skills for lecturing and supervision are not the same. Having said that, someone who is clearly interested in helping students to progress (evidenced by their willingness to handle student queries, run revision sessions, give thoughtful feedback) is likely to be conscientious in supervising their students. You should not be embarrassed to ask a potential supervisor how often he or she meets their students, nor how much time they generally take to return written work – with feedback – to a student. Ultimately, however, the best guide to their supervisory capabilities is likely to be from their current or previous students, so do make every effort to talk to them before committing yourself.

Do not assume that the more senior members of the academic staff will necessarily be the best supervisors. While it may be tempting to work with someone of international standing, you might find that you see very little of them if they spend a lot of time travelling. Senior staff may also be heavily involved in policy and administration at the institution and their time is at a premium. None of this may matter if the necessary support is available, for example, from postdoctoral assistants, but try and establish this in advance. In contrast, working with a supervisor who is relatively junior may be to your advantage – if they have not supervised many students in the past, they may feel highly committed and especially anxious to ensure their students do well. You may therefore find that you get closer supervision from a junior member of staff. The feedback from previous students will guide you here.

What sort of project will suit my skills and abilities?

You may have a clear idea about what type of project you want to do. This might be something requiring a lot of practical laboratory work, or you may prefer something that is very much 'people based'. If you enjoy statistics and data handling, you may be looking for something epidemiological. If you get satisfaction from delving into literature and synthesising a well-crafted review, then you might opt for a library or analytical project. An important part of selecting a project is choosing something where the type of work will allow you to play to your strengths. You may think you have a fair idea of your own skills and the type of things for which you show particular aptitude, but sometimes it is worth seeking external input. A student may know that he is mathematically gifted, is something of a perfectionist and pays great attention to detail, all of which would make him suited to a project that required a lot of data handling and analysis. If, however, he was someone that got frustrated if he had to rework something several times, then the project he thought would be ideal for himself might prove to be somewhat tedious.

It may be that you have already undertaken some aptitude tests as part of your course, or for other reasons. Aptitude tests are generally designed to assess abilities such as verbal reasoning, numerical reasoning, spatial reasoning and mechanical reasoning. These may provide some guidance in your choice of project. Personality tests, in contrast, provide information about such things as whether you tend to work by logic or intuition, if you prefer a structured framework or like the freedom to adapt to a changing work environment, whether you like to bounce ideas off other people, or work things out for yourself in the first instance. While these may not seem critical for your choice of **subject**, they may guide your choice of **project**. Consider the following examples:

> Melanie had always been interested in endocrinology but had never particularly enjoyed histology. She had won a prize for an essay on oestrogen, and her ultimate ambition was to work in some aspect of reproductive medicine. She knew that she got on well with people and that

she worked best in an environment where things were well ordered and not left to chance. Which of the following two projects would be the one where she would be most likely to flourish?

- Dr Black's project was based in a maternity hospital and the aim was to compare levels of progesterone in the serum of women at different stages of pregnancy. The role of the student was to collect the blood samples after the medical research fellow had taken written consent, take them to the laboratory for analysis, enter the results onto computer and relate them to questionnaire data that had been collected by the research midwife (provided that she had been available at the time of the relevant clinic visit).
- Dr Green's project was designed to look for tumour markers for bowel cancer on previously collected preserved specimens. The specimens were all available and the protocol for preparing and staining the slides, and detecting the tumour markers, was already established. The associated clinical data had been collected and was available on a computer spreadsheet.

Although Dr Black's project was in a subject area that matched Melanie's interests, she would be dependent on both the clinical research fellow and the research midwife with no certainty that the data she needed would be available. In contrast, the project offered by Dr Green had all the material available, and Melanie would not be dependent on others. Which project would best match her personal strengths?

Philip was studious and rather quiet, but could work well under pressure and planned a career in surgery. His practical skills were good and he wanted a project that would enhance his chances of a foundation year job appropriate for his ambitions.

- Dr White's project was based in a busy general practice and focused on finding out why patients sought medical advice or intervention following day-case surgery. The project included patient interviews, including assessment of their levels of satisfaction, and reviews of hospital case notes. Philip would have a lot of responsibility for the project and would have a substantial degree of independence.
- Professor Brown's project was laboratory based and looked at gastric motility in a guinea pig model. Philip would need to have an animal licence and would have a lot of 'hands-on' laboratory experience but no patient contact or overt clinical application. Professor Brown's research group was small

but close-knit, and his previous project student had enjoyed the project and done well.

Dr White's project would supply a lot of patient contact but would not provide an opportunity for using Philip's practical skills. In complete contrast, Professor Brown's project would develop these skills but the patient contact would be missing. What would you recommend Philip should do or ask about, to help him decide which project to take?

How can I know what I am letting myself in for?

Students for whom the research project is a choice rather than an integral part of their course may wonder what life will be like as a project student. Taster sessions are not likely to be available! In some ways it can be looked upon as taking a trip to a foreign land. Certain things will be strange to start with, and you will make some mistakes and get a bit lost from time to time. You may miss the comfort of a fixed routine that you share with other students, but things will gradually become familiar and at the end of the trip you will have learned a lot and have a new perspective. It is very unusual for students to withdraw from a research project once they have started: this demonstrates that almost everyone learns to cope with the transition. Talk to students who have already completed their projects and find out about their initial concerns, and ask whether their worries were unfounded. Ask about any unexpected benefits of being a project student. Try and picture yourself in the role and see if you can imagine yourself living 'a day in the life of a researcher'.

What should I do before I start?

When you know that you will be taking a research project, whether by choice or not, you can begin to prepare for it. You should familiarise yourself with all the information available to you about the research project at an early stage, from handouts, the college website and the course prospectus. The documentation about the course may be rather dry and boring, but it will answer some of the questions you may have. If anything is unclear then be prepared to ask – if you are not sure about anything, then your fellow students will probably be in the same situation! If your research project programme is one where you have spent time talking to your supervisor as part of the preliminary planning then you will already know him or her and the topic of your research. If you are assigned a supervisor, as opposed to making a choice, you will probably want to meet up before beginning work so that at least you know what he or she looks like! This may seem trivial but it can be important: someone of my acquaintance once mistook a senior member of staff for the plumber who was expected to come to fix the radiators! By meeting up with your supervisor in advance of starting your project, you can ask if there is any preparatory work you should do, such as background reading, and agree the date and time when you are expected to begin. It is also an excellent opportunity to check whether you are going to need any special permissions or documentation for your project, such as whether you need to be named on Research Ethics forms or (if you will be working with children or vulnerable adults) you need a Criminal Records Bureau (CRB) check. These can take some time to arrange, so ensuring that all is in place before you start may avoid delays when time is at a premium. Furthermore, your supervisor can be reassured that their project student is enthusiastic, forward-thinking and organised, all of which bodes well for a fruitful collaboration.

SUMMARY

Where you have a choice about taking up a research project or not, weigh up all the advantages and disadvantages, bearing in mind that your decision may affect others.

Do not assume that the project that seems (by its title) to be an ideal choice for you will necessarily be the one for which you are best suited.

Read all the guidance provided by your institution, however boring, so that you know exactly what is expected of you.

Before the project starts, meet up with your supervisor and see what preparations you can make to ensure you can 'hit the ground running'.

WHAT PROJECT CHOICES WOULD YOU RECOMMEND FOR MELANIE AND PHILIP?

There is not a crystal-clear answer to either of these dilemmas, so I can only provide a personal view. For Melanie, Dr Green's project seems a safe bet, because the material is all available and she would not be dependent on others. However, Dr Black's project may give more opportunity for Melanie to explore a range of factors affecting the serum progesterone levels – in other words, perhaps to have more 'ownership' of the project. I would advise Melanie to meet with the Medical Research Fellow and the Midwife associated with Dr Black's project. If they seemed enthusiastic, totally committed and welcomed Melanie as part of their team, then I would recommend Dr Black's project in the maternity hospital. If there were any doubts at all, I would say she should choose Dr Green's project and take the opportunity to become a proficient histologist, focus on completing the

work in a timely manner and take the initiative in preparing the work for
presentation and/or publication.

Philip's choice is equally difficult. The topic of Dr White's project would
bring a new insight into the patient's view of surgery, and this would be
valuable for the future career he planned. However, Philip is a quiet
individual and, in a busy setting in General Practice, someone with an
outgoing personality may be better at gaining collaboration from staff in the
practice and the patients, which would be essential. I would suggest
Professor Brown's project would better play to Philip's strengths (his practical
skills), and he could focus on possible clinical applications of the work in his
background reading, literature review and suggestions for ongoing research.

Chapter 2 **Getting going**

CHAPTER OVERVIEW

This chapter focuses very much on planning. It emphasises the skills you will need and the importance of keeping a record of what you have been doing. It highlights the importance of personal conduct and a professional attitude at all times, whether in a laboratory or other setting.

Introduction

Getting going can be difficult. Much depends on the individual nature of each project and the style of the supervisor. You may be plunged in at the deep end or find yourself floundering in the shallows. Your work may be very directed, or you might be left to your own devices.

Whatever is arranged for you (or not), you should make a plan. Failing to plan is like planning to fail. You will need to plan your time and your tasks. You are going to need background knowledge, practical skills, analytical skills and skills in presenting your work, orally and in writing. You may need to collect and handle lots of data. You may need to interact with many different people, colleagues and possibly patients or volunteers. Once you have established the tasks, you can think about the time frame for getting these under way. There may well be external deadlines imposed by your institution and these will affect when certain things need to be completed. Pretty soon you may want a chart to work with, which might look something like the chart shown in Figure 2.1.

Why not draw up your own chart, suitable for the project you will be working on? It may get modified over the course of the project but some

How to do your Research Project: A Guide for Students in Medicine and the Health Sciences, First Edition. Caroline Beardsmore.
© 2013 John Wiley & Sons, Ltd. Published 2013 by John Wiley & Sons, Ltd.

Diabetes and ocular problems project

Tasks	Sep	Oct	Nov	Dec	Jan	Feb	Mar	Apr	May
Courses and workshops	Induction 4–9 Sep		Intro to stats 16 Oct	Scientific writing 5 Dec	Stats part 2 14 Jan	Stats 'clinic' 11 Feb	Giving spoken presentations 21 Mar		Viva preparation 29 May
Review of literature	'Eye problems in diabetes and how to assess them'								
Write Intro & Aims									
Learn set-up & calibration									
Subject recruitment									
Practical work with subjects									
Write Methods									
Data entry and analysis					Prelim analysis				
Statistical analysis									
Write results and discussion									
Final revisions to dissertation									

Review 1, 18 Nov — Review 2, 23 Mar — Hand-in 26 MAY!

Figure 2.1 A possible project plan. This is a very broad outline but does highlight when certain aspects of the work are expected to be running. Shading has been used to link work of the same category.

things (like the hand-in date!) will not be subject to change. Getting a feel for how things might progress over the time available is very valuable. Different aspects of the project can run concurrently to make things more efficient; in Figure 2.1, for example, the subject recruitment can start while the student is still learning the experimental setup and calibration. This means that when the student is experienced enough to test the subjects, the first ones are already recruited and just need to be given an appointment. Depending on how the project progresses in the early stages, you may need to be flexible in your approach and change the plan as things develop over time. This type of chart will help you to see how your time is likely to be spent at different points in the months of the project – this student is going to be busy in December! Be realistic when making your plan, making sure that if you have other activities that you know will take you away from the workplace these are factored in. Holidays are the obvious ones, but there may be others. You will have been encouraged to maintain a healthy work–life balance during your time at medical school so far, and the time when you are a project student is no different. If you play in a sports team engaged in a knockout competition, will you expect to play if the team makes it into the final? What family events are likely to come up? If there is a party for your parents' silver wedding one Saturday and you are travelling home for that, you are unlikely to get much work done that weekend!

A plan can help you visualise the timings of the project, but you will still need to consider the tasks you must achieve. How are you going to equip yourself with all the skills you need for a great project?

Background knowledge

What basic knowledge will you need to help you achieve a really good project? You may well have the basics from earlier medical school modules. Look out your old notes and – particularly – any reading lists. Remember those reading lists – where you chose the one book that everyone else said was all you needed? Or perhaps you went to the library and borrowed the thinnest book or went to the bookshop and bought the cheapest one on the list? Well, perhaps, now is the time to get hold of all the others and read relevant sections of all of them. Authors have their strengths and weaknesses, their hobby horses and their preferences, and you will have to pick and choose. If your project is in an area that moves fast, then textbooks can quickly go out of date and you should ensure that what you are reading is not too historic to be of use. On the other hand, sometimes a broad overview is essential before you focus on an area and a clearly written introductory chapter can give you the scaffolding of knowledge to build upon.

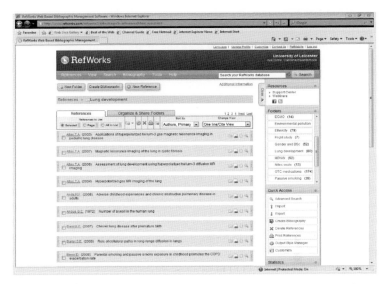

Figure 2.2 Illustration of a reference managing system. The system allows searching and importing of references directly into the electronic system, arrangement and rearrangement of references into different folders, links to the abstracts and other features. One essential feature is the ability to place numbered references in the text of any document and to produce a perfect bibliography at the end.

A good source of introductory reading is often a well-written review article in a highly ranked journal. Journal rankings are a measure of the overall quality of the journal, reflecting the impact of the work they publish (usually based on how frequently the articles are cited by other authors). Highly ranked journals reject a larger proportion of the manuscripts submitted than the lower-ranked journals. Review articles in high-ranking journals are likely to have been commissioned and should refer to all major references.

When you begin to assemble your own reading list your supervisor should be able to suggest some key references or books and point you in the right direction. You will, however, be likely to use online literature searches of established databases to build up your references. Furthermore, when it comes to writing up your dissertation, you will need to use an electronic reference managing system such as RefWorks (Figure 2.2) or EndNote. Do **not** leave this 'to be organised when you get round to it': start it on day one.

The days of typing out the references at the end of writing a dissertation or article are long gone, thank goodness. If you have not used a reference managing system before, ask if there is any training offered by your institution to help you get started, both with literature searches and the use of a reference managing system. It is likely that one of the library staff will have the responsibility for training in this area, so if such support is not laid out for you, then go and ask for it. You may like to ask around to see if other students may also benefit from such training because it is better use of time for the trainer to be working with more than one person at a time.

Conducting a literature search and being focused in your reading

Performing a literature search may be something with which you are already familiar, but you may not have had much experience and the sheer volume of published work may be daunting. As with training in the most effective use of reference management systems, your institution library may offer training in how to conduct a literature search. A good literature search should be an effective and efficient means of locating the information you need for your project. The key to this is to be very focused in defining your topic and your search terms, and your selection of databases to search.

Imagine your project is an analytical study of complications following hip replacement. If you use SCOPUS, and search for references to 'hip replacement' from 2008 to 2012 you will find 8620 hits. When these are combined with 'post-operative complications and treatment outcome', these are reduced to a more manageable 43. However, the same search strategy with Medline found just 1506 hits for 'hip replacement' alone, but 64 for the combined search terms. Repeating the search on Medline, but substituting 'hip arthroplasty' for 'hip replacement' gave 139 hits for the combined search terms. Of course the important thing is how relevant the articles are to the topic of the project, but it serves to illustrate the importance of not being too restrictive in the literature search. Having run a literature search employing your chosen key words, you may decide to restrict the search in order to make it more manageable to skim through. If our search of 139 articles is limited to adult patients, published in the English language, and restricted to medical and nursing journals only, it comes down to just 97 articles. Some of what we have cut out is information about the materials used in hip joints and their manufacture, published in journals relating to materials science and perhaps not relevant to this student project. Once you have a manageable search, then you can examine the list of articles, selecting the ones you want to read in depth. To help you do this, you can usually access the abstract of the work online, which allows you to select only those articles relevant for your work. The number of articles and the extent of your reading will be driven by the time available for your project and the type of work you are doing. If you move on at a later stage in your career to study for a PhD or an MD, you will be expected to read much more extensively than what is required for an undergraduate project of, perhaps, a few weeks or a term.

A frequent 'beginners' mistake' in literature searching is to neglect to save the search strategy. There are two reasons why this is important. First, if you want to rerun the search, perhaps using a different search engine, or to update with any recent literature, you will need it. Second, particularly with an analytical or a library project, you will need to provide the details of your research strategies. They are an essential part of your methods.

Once you have started to assemble your reading material, you need to organise what you will read, so that your reading is relevant, focused and manageable. Few people will read half a dozen papers in an evening and, of those that do, even fewer will retain the information. Be realistic about what you can cover. One way to make the most of the time you have for reading is not to get trapped into reading every section of a review or every chapter in a book. If your project is based on macrophages in the blood, you may choose to only skim the sections on macrophages in the lung. If you are working on the epidemiology of lung cancer, the details of cancer treatment (while certainly important) may not contribute to your project and might divert you from achieving your task. Having said this, there is always a tension between the breadth of knowledge and getting sufficient focus. Where you are uncertain about the extent of your background reading, discuss this with your supervisor.

Reading scientific articles is not like reading a novel or a magazine. The information you acquire by engaging with the literature in your chosen field will influence what you do and what you write. You will use it to interpret your own findings and suggest the next stages in your research. Your reading must be an active process, unlike skimming a newspaper, and the information should be retained where you can access it again as you need it. Your electronic referencing system will be invaluable here because you will be able to recall the abstracts with a few clicks of a mouse. This is not a substitute, however, for a thorough and careful reading of the sources you consult. The best way of ensuring that you have taken on board the main points of the article is to make notes as you go along or to summarise the article once you have finished reading it. In the days before ubiquitous personal computers, the usual practice was to summarise each paper on a reference card (Figure 2.3), which was then stored in a box designed for the purpose. While this may now seem a very antiquated system, the process of writing a précis of each paper you read cannot be bettered as a means of testing your understanding of what has passed from the printed page into your brain.

Making a summary or a précis of a paper is an easy skill to acquire, once you appreciate the importance of knowing why that particular publication

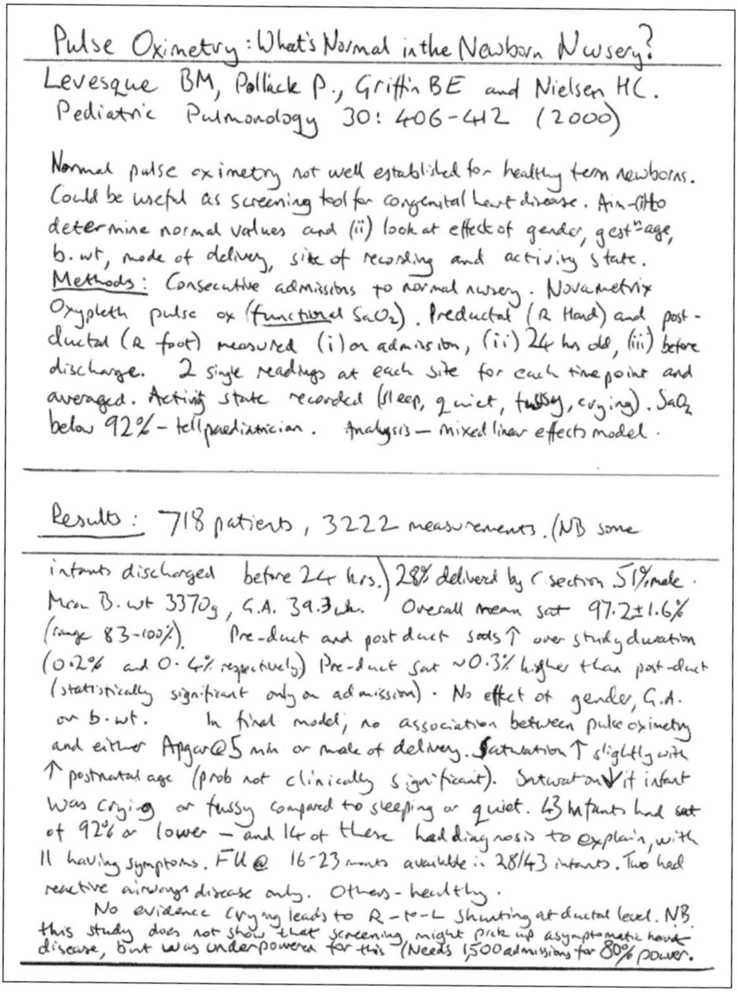

Pulse Oximetry: What's Normal in the Newborn Nursery?
Levesque BM, Pollack P., Griffin BE and Nielsen HC.
Pediatric Pulmonology 30: 406-412 (2000)

Normal pulse oximetry not well established for healthy term newborns. Could be useful as screening tool for congenital heart disease. Aim-(i) to determine normal values and (ii) look at effect of gender, gestn age, b.wt, mode of delivery, site of recording and activity state.
Methods: Consecutive admissions to normal nursery. Novametrix Oxypleth pulse ox (functional SaO_2). Preductal (R Hand) and post-ductal (R foot) measured (i) on admission, (ii) 24 hrs old, (iii) before discharge. 2 single readings at each site for each timepoint and averaged. Activity state recorded (sleep, quiet, fussy, crying). SaO_2 below 92% - tell paediatrician. Analysis — mixed linear effects model.

Results: 718 patients, 3222 measurements. (NB some infants discharged before 24 hrs.) 28% delivered by C section. 51% male. Mean B. wt 3370g, G.A. 39.3 wk. Overall mean sat 97.2±1.6% (range 83-100%). Pre-duct and post duct sats ↑ over study duration (0.2% and 0.4% respectively) Pre-duct sat ~0.3% higher than post-duct (statistically significant only on admission). No effect of gender, G.A. or b.wt. In final model, no association between pulse oximetry and either Apgar @ 5 min or mode of delivery. Saturation ↑ slightly with ↑ postnatal age (prob not clinically significant). Saturation ↓ if infant was crying or fussy compared to sleeping or quiet. 43 infants had sat of 92% or lower — and 14 of these had diagnosis to explain, with 11 having symptoms. F/U @ 16-23 months available in 28/43 infants. Two had reactive airways disease only. Others - healthy.
No evidence crying leads to R-to-L shunting at ductal level. NB this study does not show that screening might pick up asymptomatic heart disease, but was underpowered for this (Needs 1,500 admissions for 80% power.

Figure 2.3 Reference card with précised paper.

is important to you. If it is because it describes one of the techniques you will be applying, the Methods section will be prominent and you may go into some detail. If it is a publication in which the results differ from your own, you would expect to focus on any differences that could account for this and how the authors interpret their findings. Whatever the value to you of the paper you are summarising, if you restrict yourself to a single record card, rather than making notes in a book or a large file, you will force yourself to be concise and not run the risk of rewriting the whole article!

Every dissertation will include a section entitled 'Background' or 'Introduction' or 'Review of the Literature'. If you want to get ahead of the game and take the pressure off yourself as the time to submit your dissertation appears frighteningly close, you can write this (or at least a first draft) in the very early stages of your project (see Chapter 5). You may find that what you write initially undergoes several revisions, or certain parts get relocated to the 'Discussion' section in the interests of balance, but if you have written things in draft form you will find it relatively simple to work towards the final product.

Practical and laboratory skills

The practical skills needed by students doing projects can be very wide ranging. Some projects may not involve any laboratory work at all, whereas others may use highly complex 'wet laboratory' techniques, and others may be based in a hospital or other laboratory setting. Wherever you are based, you will need to be aware of the health and safety considerations.

Laboratory safety

It is likely that you will be given an introduction to the laboratory and what you will be doing when you start your project. You will almost certainly be given a copy of the laboratory safety manual to read, and you may be asked to sign to show that you have read it. If you are not asked to do this, then you should ask to see the laboratory safety manual. Safety manuals may be among the most boring things you will ever have to read, but they have been written for a purpose. You have a responsibility for your own safety, and that of others, and being the newest, most junior person in the laboratory does not absolve you from that responsibility. Some safety-related matters are so obvious they may not appear in the manual, but a moment's thought will show you why the following things are important:

- **Appropriate dress.** If a laboratory coat is mandatory, it should always be worn, and should be fastened properly and not left flapping open. Long hair should be tied back and long, dangling earrings should be left at home. Jewellery that might interfere with what you are doing should not be worn. Your shoes should be suitable. This usually means closed shoes, since any chemicals spilled on your feet will be as unpleasant as getting them on your hands. Where protective clothing is provided for specific procedures, such as goggles, aprons or masks you should always use them.

- **Nail polish.** Nail polish should be saved for social occasions because it can obscure dirty fingernails. These are certainly unacceptable in a clinical setting and undesirable in most laboratories.
- **Background music.** You may be one of the many people who like to work with background music, especially if performing a boring or repetitive task – and some laboratory tasks fall into these categories! There may be a radio or CD player in the laboratory but, if not, do ask before assuming it is acceptable to use a personal stereo. Some laboratories will allow this if only one earpiece is used, in order that the wearer can still hear if a colleague needs to call for help or shout a warning.
- **Eating and drinking.** With very few exceptions, eating, drinking and applying makeup are forbidden in laboratories, for the obvious reasons that such practices can range from the unpleasant to the frankly dangerous. They are also deeply unprofessional – and this includes the use of chewing gum.
- **Mobile telephones.** In many settings these are an unnecessary and unwelcome distraction. If a student is engaged in a phone call he or she may not be able to concentrate on the experimental work. Of course there are plenty of occasions when the mobile phone is a boon, especially if working out of a university or healthcare setting, but on a routine basis they should be switched off while you are working.
- **Personal possessions.** Personal possessions (e.g. handbags, pencil cases, laptops) may not be permitted on the laboratory bench, and if this is the case you should expect to be provided with a secure locker for your personal possessions. You may consider using a bumbag or a small bag you can wear across your body in which to keep your money or credit cards for the days you will be working in the laboratory.

During the course of your project you may find that others in the laboratory ignore or bend some of the safety guidance or rules (Figure 2.4). This may put you in a difficult situation as they are likely to be people senior to you. You should not turn a blind eye to unacceptable practices. It may not be necessary to report them for their behaviour since they may simply be unaware that they are not following the best practice. A casual remark such as 'I thought I read in the safety manual that we should always wear protective goggles when working with the Thingummybob Machine?' might be all that is required.

Conduct in a clinical setting

Many students prefer a clinically-based project to a more traditional laboratory-based project, especially if they are at an early stage in their medical school career and want to get into a clinical environment. In this situation, the student is likely to be interacting with other healthcare workers as well as patients or volunteer subjects and possibly their relatives. If this is your

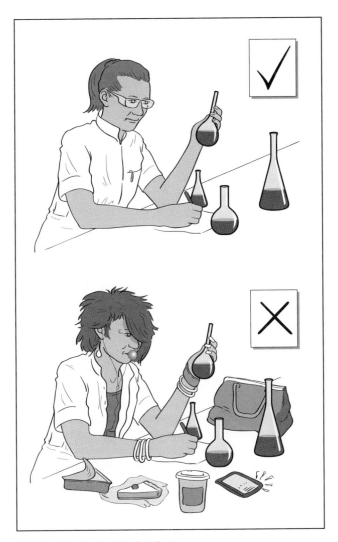

Figure 2.4 Good student and bad student.

choice, everyone you work alongside will expect you to behave in a professional manner. Patients, in particular, may see you as someone with authority and knowledge, and this may place you in a different situation to your fellow student who is laboratory based. The dress code is likely to be the same as for any of your clinical placements, that is, 'clean and neat and tidy', and if you are unsure whether something is too casual or not, then it probably is! Check in advance whether you will be expected to wear a white coat or not, and if you need to provide this yourself make sure it is clean and ironed. Senior police officers who do not wear uniform are advised to dress in a manner so that anyone they may interview would find it hard to recall what they were wearing! This might be overly strict for the medical profession, but there is some merit in this advice. You will be expected to wear an identification badge at all times. If yours has got a bit grubby, use an Alcowipe or cloth soaked in a dilute cleaning fluid to restore it to a pristine condition.

Your supervisor is likely to introduce you to colleagues and those working in your clinical setting, and do try to get to know their various roles and responsibilities. Do not be shy about telling them what your project is all about because they may be able to make suggestions or observations that will be invaluable. They are likely to know the patients in their ward or clinic and may be able to smooth the path for you.

Occasionally, a student project may be conducted away from a university or the usual healthcare setting, perhaps because it involves visiting patients in their own homes. Visiting someone's home should be seen as a privilege, and you should be sensitive towards their lifestyle and the needs of the patient and the other members of the family. Conducting an interview may take much longer than you anticipate. Someone who is housebound may lack company and want to chat about matters unrelated to your research, or a mother of young children may have to break off to attend to their needs. Use these opportunities to build a rapport with the patient and to reflect on the impact of the medical condition you are researching on everyday life. If you are working away from your medical school or hospital, your own safety should be considered. Make sure that someone connected to your project knows exactly where you are going and at what time, and when you expect to leave. A system of telephoning to report the conclusion of a visit may be appropriate. Although it is rare, it is not unknown for healthcare workers to be threatened (or to feel threatened) in the course of their work. You should not put yourself in a situation where you are at any risk. If you do find yourself in such a situation, you should make a suitable excuse and leave, and report to your supervisor at the earliest opportunity.

Ethical aspects of clinical research

Before any work on a clinical research project starts, it requires approval from a Research Ethics Committee. It also requires a sponsor, frequently an NHS Trust. This means that the sponsor has agreed to support the research done on their premises and to indemnify it. The research study should have a site file, which contains all the paperwork relating to the study (ethics committee applications, protocols, details of funding, copies of information sheets, consent forms, correspondence, etc.) and you should know where this file is kept. Looking at the mountains of paperwork in the site file will give you an appreciation of how much preparation goes into clinical research before any human volunteer is approached. You should ask for copies of the approval letters and any other relevant documents so that you can include them in your dissertation, most likely in an appendix. Your supervisor should know if the regulatory bodies require notification that you have joined the research project, and in this case your name needs to be added to the list of people involved, which is part of the site file. There is no harm in checking with your supervisor whether this needs to be done because it is the type of thing that could easily get overlooked!

Because of the amount of work required for a study involving human subjects to be approved by a Research Ethics Committee, it is unlikely that many students are required to work with the online forms that are a part of the Integrated Research Application System (IRAS), or indeed to have knowledge of the Health Research Authority (HRA) that has the responsibility for the National Research Ethics Service. Nevertheless, it is worth spending some time exploring the HRA website in order to see the extent of planning that is required by the regulatory authorities. Until you become involved in clinical research, your knowledge and experience of medical ethics is likely to have come from parts of the medical curriculum where you have been asked to consider the ethical aspects of the right to die, issues surrounding termination of pregnancy, rights of patients to refuse treatment, importance of confidentiality and the circumstances when this may be broken, decisions on healthcare rationing and many other issues that challenge the medical profession. You may not have had the opportunity to consider the ethics surrounding medical research, which is a subject in itself. The World Medical Association made their Declaration of Helsinki in 1964, which sets down the principles that underpin medical research. These have been refined and published in different guises over the intervening years, and a basic understanding of the guiding principles, as set out in a bulletin of the World Health Organisation, will help your understanding of research ethics. Specific guidelines are available for certain categories of patients or volunteers; for example, the Royal College of Paediatrics and Child Health publish guidelines on the ethical conduct of medical research involving children.

When working with human subjects, the key principles for ethical conduct of research include the taking of consent. Consent can only be given by someone who is competent to do so; that is, they have the capacity to understand fully what they are asked to consider. They should be provided with all the information relevant to their participation, and consent should be freely and voluntarily given. As a student, you may not be taking formal (written) consent from your subjects, but you may well be in the position of talking about the research to volunteers and patients. You have a duty to provide information in an unbiased manner with no element of coercion. This may seem tough when you are keen to recruit the target number of subjects and when (in your opinion) what you are asking is not onerous. Although many people are altruistic and willing to help in research, remember that others may have a very different view of what is acceptable to them, no doubt influenced by their culture, emotions and previous experiences. You might want to think about all possible reasons why someone might choose **not** to get involved in your project, by asking family and friends (especially those with no medical background) why they might decline to participate. Box 2.1 gives an example of how this might turn out.

Box 2.1 Reasons for not participating in a particular research project

Imagine a project is designed to look at the links between physical fitness and blood cholesterol levels in young adults. The plan is to work with healthy volunteers, recruited from the student halls of residence and the student sports centre. You anticipate each volunteer will have an appointment of 1 hour, to include completion of a questionnaire on lifestyle and fitness, followed by giving a small blood sample and an exercise test on a treadmill while you record heart rate, speed and slope of treadmill and time to exhaustion. Make a list of possible reasons why someone would **not** take part.

The first two points are fairly obvious, but later ones may not have occurred to you:

- Needle phobia – no chance of getting blood
- Too busy – exams coming up
- Fear of the cholesterol test – what if they had a very high reading? (i) Would it mean they had a risk of heart disease? (ii) Would it affect their life insurance policy?
- Embarrassment about the questionnaire – what if there are questions about sexual activity?
- Subject is on long-term medication and would not want to disclose the reasons for this
- Subject is worried that she may be pregnant and is concerned about the possible effect of the test
- Subject hates running and would not want to get red, hot and sweaty in front of others

You may feel that the last reason is completely unreasonable and that the importance of your project far outweighs it, but the potential volunteer has a different viewpoint and you must accept the validity of this.

If your project is one in which you will want to recruit healthy controls, you might assume that you will ask all your medical student friends to volunteer. Your medical school may have guidance on participation of students in research because there is the possibility that their participation is partly coerced (e.g. fear of being given a poor grade by a member of staff if they do not volunteer), so you should check the circumstances under which their involvement is permitted.

Learning the practical skills

It is likely that you will need to be shown some new skills for your project. These may be so-called wet laboratory skills that could involve complex things such as cell culture, microdissection, chromatography, nerve conduction experiments – you name it; someone will have to show you what to do. Some individuals are natural teachers and you will quickly grasp what you need to know and do. When this is not the case, you will need to be proactive in your own learning. For example, if you watch someone do something you may remember seeing it done, but if you do something yourself you are much more likely to be able to do it again correctly the next time. Ask the person showing you a new technique if you can have a go yourself, and if he or she will watch you. Make sure you understand what it is you are trying to do. If it is something that requires practice, perhaps you can gain this by offering to help someone else in the laboratory for the purposes of gaining experience.

Many laboratory techniques are described in Standard Operating Procedures (SOPs), and you may be provided with SOPs that you will need. It is a good idea to have someone around when using an SOP for the first time, in case something that should be clear turns out not to be! If there are no SOPs for the techniques you will be using, then why not offer to write them for your laboratory? This will ensure that you have them written down precisely – what a good start for when you want to write up the Methods section of your project! In addition to following (or writing) an SOP, you may find it very helpful to take a digital camera into the laboratory to photograph the equipment and/or the experimental set-up you use. A photograph or two can certainly help an SOP and, again, will be invaluable when it comes to illustrating your Methods section.

Your laboratory project may require certain disposable items or single-use equipment or reagents with limited shelf life. These will add to the costs of running your project. Find out what your project will cost; you will probably be shocked! You may be able to minimise the costs by careful planning of your work; for example, if a bottle of one of your reagents lasts 3 days after opening, can you arrange to bring it into use early in the week and avoid needing a new bottle on a Friday? Can you share things with others in the laboratory to cut costs? Careful financial management of the project will not only go down well with your supervisor but if your experimental work is constrained by costs you may be able to extend your project by conserving and managing your resources. Your supervisor is more likely to offer you the opportunity to do some vacation work if he or she can see that you are aware of the costs of research.

Any laboratory procedure will generate a certain amount of clearing up and cleaning of equipment, and possibly storage of samples. You should take the responsibility for this and not assume others will do it for you. By taking responsibility for the equipment, you will become more familiar with it and this will enhance your learning. Your supervisor may have a research technician who will take care of these 'housekeeping' tasks for some of the laboratory work, but it does not follow automatically that he or she will do the same for a student doing a project. Find out what is expected of you and be prepared to volunteer to share the load of the unglamorous laboratory tasks. Some of the processes may result in the need to dispose of chemicals, biological samples such as blood or urine, or possibly laboratory animals that have been sacrificed. Make sure that you know the correct route for disposing of anything you will be using because the wrong route of disposal may have severe consequences for the laboratory. When you are leaving preparations such as agar plates in a temperature-controlled environment or storing samples in the laboratory freezer make sure the items are clearly and sensibly labelled so that others will recognise that they are important. Putting your name and the date of storage clearly on your samples in indelible marker will be a good start. Someone tasked with 'clearing out the laboratory freezer' is unlikely to dispose of samples marked 'Urine from diabetic patients (study # 6-12) – stored 3/4/2010 by Jake Smith', but something labelled simply 'Jakes Urine' might find its way into the nearest sewer.

Keeping a laboratory book/log book

A laboratory book is documentary evidence of your work. It is a permanent record of what you have done, why and how you did it, what results you obtained and your plans for the future. It is a very important document that should allow any other scientist to follow exactly what you did with no space for doubt. A laboratory book can be used as evidence (e.g. if you are taking out a patent and need to demonstrate that you were the first person to design and use a particular piece of apparatus) and as such it needs be robust.

It is something that should be left behind in the laboratory after you have completed your project and left.

Files for loose sheets of paper or ring-bound books should not be used because of the potential for removing bits of paper without any trace. Paper should never be torn from your laboratory book because you could always be challenged about what might be missing. Laboratory books should be hard bound and of a type that makes it impossible for sheets to be torn out without trace. For similar reasons, all the entries in the laboratory book should be in a pen that cannot be erased, and never in pencil. When you make mistakes, these should be lightly crossed out by pen and the revised version written alongside or above the original entry.

Your laboratory book will need to be identifiable as yours, so write your name prominently on the cover and ensure your contact details can be easily found. It is probably worth noting your supervisor's name as well, and the location to which the book should be returned if it is found somewhere such as the cafeteria or cloakroom of your building. Some supervisors insist on the laboratory books remaining in the laboratory (usually in a secure location) where they can access them at any time. If this is the case in your setting, you may wish to take photocopies of certain parts for your private use and records.

It is useful to have a book with numbered pages and to leave the first couple of pages for a table of contents because you may organise the book into different sections. For example, you may keep a section near the back for names and addresses of suppliers of equipment and reagents. The bulk of your laboratory book will be something like a diary or journal because you will be recording what you do on a day-to-day basis. For this reason every entry should be dated. You should include the basis for your experimental work as well as the details of your experiments. In entering the details of your experiments, there may be occasions when you reference SOPs but you should be meticulous in noting down any additional details that could influence the results. The SOP for your experiment on the rat kidney may be excellent, but you will still need to record the species of rat, its age, sex, weight, anaesthetic agent and dose and anything else that may be relevant. This type of information should be directly recorded in the laboratory book, along with any observations about the experiment or deviations from protocol. Your results should also be in your laboratory book. These may be handwritten, or in the form of a printout, a photograph or a combination (Figure 2.5). Where they come as a separate item, this must be secured in the laboratory book and not just tucked in between pages from where it will inevitably fall out. The results should be annotated and the implications written down at the time, perhaps with suggestions for future work.

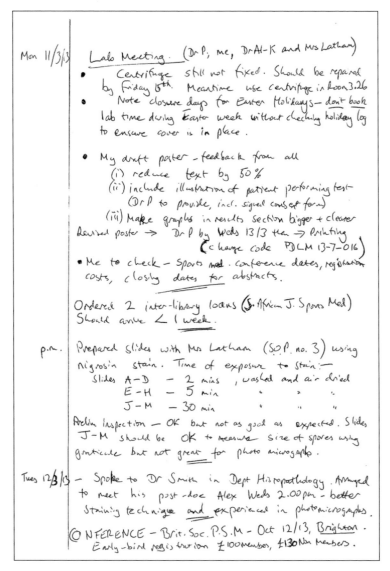

Figure 2.5 Example of a page from a laboratory book.

You may be wondering why, in the twenty-first century, you are not being encouraged to keep a digital laboratory book and keep everything electronically. There are several reasons. It is often easier to jot down a few thoughts in a book, and definitely easier to make a quick sketch, than to attempt this on a laptop or similar device. You cannot readily stick certain specialist print-outs onto a laptop. By dating every entry, you will find it easier to maintain a chronological record. Most importantly, electronic entries can usually be altered without trace, whereas a written record cannot. Having said this, you will almost certainly be using a variety of electronic formats in the course of your project and in the production of your dissertation, so, in parallel with your hard copy laboratory book, you may also want to begin an electronic collection of results tables, figures, photographs that can be readily slotted in to your *magnum opus*.

Working hours and setting your own timetable

As a project student, it is likely that you will have a lot of flexibility in your timetable, particularly in the time allocated for writing up. If you have been following a routine medical school curriculum for 2 or 3 years before your project, this will come as quite a shock to the system! Some students find it quite disconcerting and have difficulty adjusting to the change. This is when planning is really essential. Even though you are not being paid to do your project, if you approach it as you would a salaried position, then you will find it easier to keep on task and keep the work in proportion. If you were paying someone to do your project, you would expect them to be working for the hours you had negotiated and you would feel cheated if they did not. If you do not devote time and energy to your own project, the person you are cheating is chiefly yourself. Alternatively, you might find that your project begins to dominate your life totally and this is equally undesirable. Again, if you were paying someone to do your project, you might be happy for him or her to take on some unpaid overtime but you would be worried if they never had any time off!

Your working hours in the laboratory may not be set for you and will depend on myriads of factors. If you will be working independently most of the time, you may be able to come and go largely at your own convenience. If your work involves the use of shared equipment you may need to book time on this, or at least negotiate with other users when you will have time allocated. If, on the other hand, the nature of your work is such that you do not work exclusively to your own timetable, you will need to liaise with others, including fellow students, your supervisor, technical staff, PhD students, postdoctoral researchers and many others. You will need to have a flexible approach, and may need to modify your overall plan as the work progresses. Find out when you are expected to be in the laboratory from the start of your project. If you are planning the start of your own work, try to arrange things so that a member of staff is not obliged to stay late in the day because you were late starting. If the work generally begins at a given time, you should be there at the start of the working day. You are likely to find that the paid laboratory staff are much more willing to help a student if he or she turns up on time and shows enthusiasm and willingness to help than one who rolls in halfway through the morning. Similarly, a student who is prepared to stay late because a particular procedure or experiment is overrunning is going to generate more goodwill than one who disappears as soon as his or her particular experiment is complete. The enthusiastic student, moreover, is likely to learn much more than the one who focuses on their own project exclusively and does not share in the wider work and vision of their laboratory. On the days or times when you do not expect to be in the laboratory, it is a good practice to make sure your supervisor and possibly other colleagues know where you will be and how to get hold of you. Do not assume that any absences or persistent lateness on your part will go unnoticed or unremarked: even if your supervisor is not in the laboratory on a frequent or regular basis, he or she is likely to ask other colleagues how you have been getting along.

A common finding among many researchers is the feeling of having been very busy but not managing to achieve much! This can usually be attributed to poor time management. Keeping a daily log of how your time is spent, over a week, will help you identify where the time is going and what is preventing you from achieving where you want to get to (Box 2.2).

Setting your own timetable brings with it the responsibility to reach your own interim goals or milestones. When you are at the planning stage you should have flagged up the dates by which you expect to have achieved certain goals. Some of these are not entirely within your control, such as learning and practising a new technique when you need a skilled technician to show you what to do and then observe your performance. If the technician is off sick, this may be postponed. Under these circumstances the unmotivated or irresponsible student might decide to stay at home. The more proactive student might ask if there was something he or she could be doing so that the sick colleague did not return to vast amounts of work that would delay the training session still more. Another approach would be to bring forward a task scheduled for a future date, such as a literature search, that might therefore get finished ahead of the planned date.

Box 2.2   Possible log of how time was spent in an average week

Make a list of the activities you undertake during the course of a working day. Be honest, and include things that are peripheral to your project or, indeed, unrelated to it. Then fill in a daily log of what you spend your time doing. It might resemble the table below.

	Mon	Tue	Wed	Thu	Fri
09:00	E-mails	Set-up and	Meet with	Set-up and	Wrote part of
09:30	Set up and	calibration	supervisor	calibration	the literature
10:00	calibrated	Measurement	Lit search and	Measurements	review
10:30	equipment	with patient 1	downloading	with patient 2	
11:00	Sent out information		manuscripts		E-mails
11:30	sheets to patients	Cleaning equipment	E-mails	Waiting – patient 3 did not come	Helped Mandy with her experiments
12:00	Design and print	E-mails	Reading and making notes for literature review	E-mails	
12:30	BBQ tickets	Lunch		Measurements with control 3	Went to gym
13:00	Lunch	Measurements		Clearing up	
13:30	E-mails	with controls 1 and 2	Lunch	Lunch with Maggie	Lunch
14:00	Workshop		Helped Mandy with her experiments		Went to clinic, recruited 3
14:30				Wrote part of literature review	patients
15:00		Clearing up	Telephoned controls to confirm attendance		E-mails
15:30			Took photos of experimental set-up for Methods section	Sent information sheets to patients	
16:00	Trial run of	Journal club	Football		
16:30	measurements on self			Departmental seminar	Shopping for BBQ, went home
17:00	Cleaning equipment	Met Jools to plan BBQ			
17:30	Went home	Went home			
18:00				Went to pub	

Note that only 6 hours were spent making measurements with patients or controls, but the student found 2 hours to help another student with her experiments. Six hours were devoted to the literature review, but $3^1/_2$ hours were devoted to e-mails (how many of these were work related?). However, the log indicates how much time needs to be spent on setting up and calibrating equipment, and clearing up after experimental work, and presumably these cannot be reduced.

SUMMARY

Failing to plan is like planning to fail.

Work out what background knowledge you will need and organise your reading to acquire this. Use a reference managing system from day one.

Spend some time considering the ethical and research governance aspects of your work. This is true even if your project does not involve you with direct laboratory work or interactions with patients or volunteers.

If you are working in a laboratory setting, make sure you are aware of the health and safety requirements.

Keep a laboratory book or a log book of all your activities.

You are likely to have a lot of responsibility for setting your own timetable. Use your time wisely, and consider a weekly log to see how you spend this precious resource.

Further reading

Emanuel, E.J. (ed.) (2008) *The Oxford Textbook of Clinical Research Ethics*, Oxford University Press.

Haynes, M.E. (2000) *Make Every Minute Count*, 3rd edn, Kogan Page.

World Health Organisation (2001)World Medical Association declaration of Helsinki: ethical principles for medical research involving human subjects. Bulletin of the World Health Organisation, 79 (4), 373.

The following websites give useful suggestions on how to keep a laboratory log book:

http://www3.imperial.ac.uk/pls/portallive/docs/1/7289716.PDF (last accessed 14 January 2013).

http://home.clara.net/rod.beavon/lab_book.htm (last accessed 14 January 2013)

The Health Research Authority website provides information and guidance on getting Research Ethics Committee approval for research involving human subjects:

http://www.hra.nhs.uk/ (last accessed 14 January 2013)

Chapter 3 **The supervisor and other colleagues**

CHAPTER OVERVIEW

This chapter discusses the roles and responsibilities of different people you may work alongside for the duration of your project and the importance of good working relationships. Recognising your own strengths and weaknesses, and those of others, will help you make effective progress with your project.

Your supervisor

Your supervisor is most likely to be a member of the academic staff and to have the overall responsibility for the place where you will be working (laboratory or other facility) and for supervising your work. The supervisor may also have the responsibility for securing research grant money to underpin their research programme, not to mention their teaching and any administrative or clinical commitments and the supervision of other students. The extent of these commitments will affect the time any supervisor can devote to their research project students. Additionally, supervisors will have their own preferred ways of working. Despite this, there may be institutional guidelines about how frequently and at what time points supervisors should meet with their students. Unless the guidelines are very explicit, students should ask their supervisors about their preferred ways of working. This would include nature and frequency of supervision meetings, how and when written work should be handed in, and what type of feedback can be expected. You should also establish which other people (if any) will be involved in your supervision.

Depending on the practice of the research project programme at your institution, your supervisor may have chosen to offer a research project in the hope

---

How to do your Research Project: A Guide for Students in Medicine and the Health Sciences,
First Edition. Caroline Beardsmore.
© 2013 John Wiley & Sons, Ltd. Published 2013 by John Wiley & Sons, Ltd.

Table 3.1 Contributions made by the supervisor and the student to a good working relationship during the research project

The supervisor	The student
Academic support	Motivation
Training (practical and scientific methods)	Commitment
Reviewing written work	Dedication
Providing feedback	Background knowledge and
Reporting on your progress	understanding
Involved in marking and assessment	Willingness to ask questions
Careers advice	Unafraid to challenge orthodoxy
Pastoral support	

of attracting a bright and enthusiastic student to work with. Alternatively, they may have had to offer a project as a part of their professional duties. The supervisors might be obliged to accept students for projects, whether or not they would otherwise want to recruit them. In Chapter 1, we discussed the situation in which a student may have some choice of project and supervisor, or may be allocated randomly or in some other way. Similarly, the supervisors may have some choice in which student(s) works with them, or they may have to take whoever is allocated. This might influence how they **feel** about supervising a project, but whatever system is used to bring you together should not affect the nature and quality of the supervision you receive. Whether you came together with an element of choice, or by other circumstances, you should aim to make the working relationship as productive as possible. Along with tangible resources (e.g. laboratory facilities), the supervisor will be bringing their knowledge and experience to the partnership. As the student, you can bring your own contributions, which are every bit as important (Table 3.1). By recognising what you can contribute, and demonstrating this to your supervisor, you can help build a synergistic working relationship that is a foundation for a successful project.

Professional, but friendly

Relationships between supervisors and research students are as varied as the individuals concerned. As with any relationship, it is forged by the two people involved and may change over the time you work together. Aim to contribute to a relationship that is professional, but friendly. You have come together for the purposes of the research project and that is at the heart of the collaboration. Your exchanges may relate exclusively to the project, especially if it is of a short duration or if it is a library project. If your project extends over a longer period or if you are doing practical work in your supervisor's laboratory, you are likely to get to know each other better. You will recognise that your supervisor has a life outside the workplace. Some people prefer not to discuss their friends, families or social activities in the workplace, whereas others are more talkative. Without being intrusive, you may acknowledge some aspects of the other roles of your supervisor, for example, by wishing them a good holiday or a Christmas break. If your supervisor or colleague suffers bereavement during your time as a student, it is entirely appropriate to express your condolences. If they have had some time off for a sick leave, tell them you are pleased to see they have recovered. After all, if you go back to college or university after being ill, you would think it rather strange if nobody asked you how you were feeling!

Some supervisors will take the trouble to get to know their students beyond how well they perform their research project. If you face any difficulties in other areas of your life that affect your work, then making your supervisor aware of the problem allows him or her to make allowances. For example, if you are a victim or a witness to a crime and therefore will have to go to court to give evidence, make sure your supervisor knows that you will be absent at short notice. If you are dyslexic, tell your supervisor and explain how this affects your work. If you are diabetic and need to eat at regular times or, on occasion, you need to eat something rapidly to avoid hypoglycaemia, let your supervisor know so that they do not get the wrong impression and conclude that you find lunch more important than work!

Many students will ask their supervisor to write them a reference at some point, and some may want to stay longer with their supervisor, perhaps as a PhD student or while working in some other capacity. Whatever your plans for the next stage of your studies or career, or even if you are uncertain of your next steps, it makes sense to talk to your supervisor and ask their advice. They may be able to offer suggestions that you had not thought about or be in a position to help in other ways. If you think that you may want a reference at some point in the future, you could ask your supervisor if they would prepare a reference for you towards the end of your project. In this way the reference is likely to be more accurate and reflective than something they may write several months after you have moved on to something else.

Working as part of a team

It is extremely unusual for scientists or academic staff to work in isolation, so during your project you could find yourself working alongside many people or, possibly, just one or two others. You will, however, become part of a team, even if the team comprises just you and your supervisor. This may present you with an apparent conundrum: your project needs to be your own piece of work, yet you are collaborating with others. In most cases this should not become an issue provided that all the members of the team acknowledge the collaborative nature of the research and all are prepared to support each other. Think of it as sharing a vegetable plot: before you joined the team, others had established the plot and some of the work was already under way. Within the team, there may be a head gardener who decides what needs to be done and who might take on each task, but everyone shares in the produce. Your main project might be to grow the courgettes. Someone else may need to show you what to do and give you some help, but eventually you will have some courgettes to enter into the local produce show (equivalent to handing in your dissertation). Alongside growing your courgettes, you may be asked to help plant the potatoes, water the tomatoes, thin out the lettuces, turn over the compost heap and numerous other tasks. When you are away, somebody else may look after your courgettes for you. Ultimately, everyone benefits from the whole garden by all having a share in all the vegetables. You may get most of the credit for the courgettes, but you will have gained much more than that if each member of the team has contributed unselfishly to the whole enterprise. So it is with research.

Difficulties can arise when different members of the team have different expectations. Also, since research projects vary in their timescale and nature from one institution to another, the extent to which the student can share in the overall research output will vary. Research projects that are of a short duration and where the student contribution is limited may not, for example, provide an opportunity for the student to co-author a publication. (To extend the analogy above, you may leave with a couple of courgettes but do not expect to go home with a big box of different vegetables!) What you need to do is to make it clear to your supervisor at the outset that you are keen to gain as much experience as possible from your project and willing to help with the wider work of the team or laboratory in which you are placed. You can also ascertain what you can expect in return for your hard work and commitment, perhaps by asking about the achievements of previous project students.

Something you may want to discuss is ownership of any data you may generate. In most cases it will belong to your institution. You will be using it in the course of writing up your project, but ultimately the data (whether in an electronic format or written in a laboratory book or stored in a filing cabinet) belong to your university or college and should be left with your supervisor. You may be allowed to keep a copy.

Roles and responsibilities of other members of the team

Research assistants or associates
Research assistants are frequently referred to as 'postdocs', which is short for postdoctoral research assistant or postdoctoral research fellow. The postdoc is

likely to be someone who completed their PhD fairly recently (within the last 3 years) and is consolidating their experience and skills with a view to moving into a more permanent post, though not necessarily in an academic setting. The career opportunities for postdocs will depend to some extent on their areas of expertise and some may take a series of contracts as research assistants before moving on to a different stage in their careers. Within a research setting, they will be doing a lot of the 'hands-on' work, but providing substantial intellectual input into experimental planning and data interpretation as well.

Technical staff

Technicians are usually employed to undertake much of the day-to-day work of the laboratory, although their roles may extend far beyond this. A few may have permanent posts, but many will be working on a contract. In some cases a technician will have worked for several years in one department, funded in a series of contracts. It is increasingly rare to find laboratory technicians who do not have a university degree, and some may have a master's degree or occasionally a doctorate. Some people fund their postgraduate studies by working as technicians, so you may be working alongside a technician who is also registered as a student. The levels of qualification and experience within the technical workforce vary tremendously. Their work may be very varied, as they may be involved in providing support for undergraduate practical classes, or in providing a clinical service, along with their role in supporting research. They are likely to be involved in maintaining equipment, ordering consumables and things such as keeping a record of laboratory safety checks as well as experimental work.

There may be considerable overlap of roles and responsibilities between research assistants and technical staff. Historically, a technician was not expected to make a major intellectual contribution to a research programme in the way that was expected of a research assistant, but this distinction has become increasingly blurred. If you find yourself working with research assistants and/or technical staff, you may find that they will both be involved in supervising you on a day-to-day basis and in helping you learn the skills and techniques you need for your project.

Graduate students

Graduate students will be registered for a second degree, which could be at the Master's level (Master of Science (MSc) or Master of Philosophy (MPhil)) or at the doctoral level (Doctor of Medicine (MD) or Doctor of Philosophy (PhD)). The term 'philosophy', when used in the context of MPhil or PhD does not imply that the students are working in the discipline of philosophy, poring over the works of Kant, Aristotle, Descartes and others. It is simply the manner of indicating the level of study in which the student is engaged and not the topic of study.

MSc students usually work full-time for a year or part-time over 2 years, although there may be local variations. Typically, they have some taught courses and a research project. MPhil students will usually spend 2 years on a research project, although they may have some taught components as well. The duration of a doctoral degree will vary, in part, according to whether the student is registered full-time or part-time. Typically, a full-time PhD student will spend 3–4 years performing their programme of research and writing their thesis. MD students will already be qualified medical doctors who are choosing to spend some time (usually 2–4 years) on a medical research project. To add to the confusion, although MD is a higher degree in the United Kingdom, you may find medical doctors who have graduated from countries where MD is the name given to the basic medical qualification. Whatever the name of the degrees for which the graduate students are registered, they are likely to be working in areas related to your own and may therefore be in a position to help or advise you, depending on the extent of their own experience.

Other support staff
The contribution of library staff to your research project cannot be underestimated. If you have a practical project, you will need to carry out a literature search and, in the course of writing your dissertation, you will need to place your work in context (see Chapter 5 for more details). If you are writing an extended review or your project is library based, you will be searching a range of sources, both in print and electronic. Library staff are experts in this and will be able to give you advice and help as you embark on the great sea of literature. Unless specific training sessions are organised for you at the start of your project, it is probably worth starting your literature search independently, so that you have a feel for 'what is out there' and then consulting a librarian for their advice on what you have been doing and where else you could search. Do remember to keep notes of any search strategy you may have developed, so the librarian can see what you have done and what areas remain unexplored. You might think that your literature search on a particular drug is complete, but your librarian colleague might suggest contacting the pharmaceutical company for some of the information that they hold on file, if it seems relevant to your work.

If your work is based in a hospital or other healthcare facility, you will almost certainly be working alongside medical, nursing or paramedical staff. These people may be employed specifically on a research project because of their specific skills or qualifications. For example, a drug trial may employ a research nurse who will be involved in recruiting patients to the trial, screening them for their suitability, making physiological measurements (e.g. blood pressure and ECG) and taking blood samples for laboratory tests. Alternatively, they may have only a small involvement, such as identifying patients who are due to attend an outpatient clinic and may be suitable for the specific research project. They may be doing this out of goodwill rather than as a part of their routine employment but, even if their contribution is modest, they are a part of the team. Do not forget to make sure they know who you are and what you are doing. Let them know of your progress, and acknowledge their help in any successes. Feeling that they are part of a team is important for engendering ongoing help and support.

Your team is likely to include others, even if they may play a more peripheral role. The host department will have administrative and secretarial staff who may be instrumental in sorting out your office and computer consumables, ID badges, letters of introduction and possibly the arrangements for examination of your dissertation. In many cases, these individuals will have fulfilled these roles for previous generations of project students and therefore can be a source of advice and encouragement.

Working as a member of a team

As a student doctor or a healthcare professional, you will have already experienced working in a group or a team. In many situations you will have been allocated to a group of approximately 6–10 other students and expected to work together, usually on designated tasks or with specific learning objectives in mind. On other occasions, you may have had an element of choice in who you work alongside. Whatever process is used to delineate the group or the team, you are likely to have observed that some groups work harmoniously and others seem to generate a lot of conflict. Some complete the designated tasks effectively, while others struggle. No doubt, you will have experienced frustrations with groups of which you have been part, perhaps because some members do not contribute to the work, or do not communicate effectively. Personality clashes can seriously affect the effectiveness of a group.

Some large organisations employ psychometric testing as a part of their recruitment strategy. Psychometric tests can assess a range of attributes including intelligence (itself difficult to define, as it includes diverse things such as verbal reasoning, spatial visualisation and numerical skills) and personality types. You may be familiar with some of the literature on personality types and on how to define them, and indeed you may have been tested yourself. One of the best known is the Myers-Briggs Type Indicator, which considers the functions of thinking, feeling, sensing and intuition and whether the individual expresses these in an introvert or extravert manner.

The personality type may indicate the preference of the individual (e.g. career choice), but not their ability to perform well in any particular job or role. This has been addressed in recent decades using methods developed by Meredith Belbin, widely used in management consultancy. The contribution of Belbin and his colleagues was to recognise that successful teams included individuals with different preferred roles who, when working in a team, complimented each other. Individuals can be described according to the team role they prefer to adopt, with a team role being defined as 'a tendency to behave, contribute and interrelate with others in a particular way' (http://www.belbin.com/). Nine such team roles are recognised (Table 3.2), and individuals display all these roles to a greater or lesser extent. It is perfectly possible for an individual to be both a strong coordinator and a resource investigator. Alongside each role are the 'allowable weaknesses', which are the more negative aspects of each role that tend to accompany the strengths. The important thing for successful teams is that they should be balanced so that all the roles are represented, without gaps in any team role or an excess of one Belbin type.

When you join your research team, you are most unlikely to be subjected to any kind of psychometric test or have your preferred team role evaluated. However, as you observe your colleagues, you will recognise some of their individual strengths and weaknesses in the workplace. If you can make reasonable allowances for their shortcomings you are less likely to be frustrated. For example, if your supervisor has a habit of being late for meetings, make sure you have some reading matter with you while you sit and wait. If he or she seems to have a new idea every day to add to your project, ask them at the end of the week exactly which of the brilliant ideas you need to follow up and which can be shelved – perhaps for another student next year. Similarly, an understanding of how your behaviour is perceived by others should help you settle into a new working environment. If your housemates complain about your untidiness, you should make an effort not to exhibit this negative characteristic when sharing workspace with colleagues.

Meetings

The nature and the frequency of meetings may well vary from one student placement to another. The meetings may be one-to-one meetings with your supervisor, or may include other members of the team. You may be expected – or invited – to attend other meetings, such as a departmental journal club. The format and degree of formality may vary tremendously between meetings.

At the outset of your project, you should ask about the meetings you are expected to or encouraged to attend, whether these are individual meetings specifically about your project or for your wider learning. Some meetings

Table 3.2 Belbin team roles, showing the contribution of each role and the allowable weaknesses

Role name	Team-role contribution	Allowable weaknesses
Plant	Creative, imaginative, unorthodox Solves difficult problems	Ignores incidentals Too preoccupied with own thoughts to communicate effectively
Resource investigator	Extrovert, enthusiastic, communicative Explores opportunities Develops contacts	Over-optimistic Can lose interest once initial enthusiasm has passed
Coordinator	Mature, confident Clarifies goals Brings other people together to promote team discussions	Can be seen as manipulative Offloads personal work
Shaper	Challenging, dynamic, thrives on pressure Has the drive and courage to overcome obstacles	Prone to provocation Liable to offend others
Monitor evaluator	Serious minded, strategic and discerning Sees all options Judges accurately	Can lack drive and ability to inspire others
Teamworker	Cooperative, mild, perceptive and diplomatic Listens, builds, averts friction	Indecisive in crunch situations
Implementer	Disciplined, reliable, conservative in habits A capacity for taking practical steps and actions	Somewhat inflexible Slow to respond to new possibilities
Completer finisher	Painstaking, conscientious, anxious Searches out errors and omissions Delivers on time	Inclined to worry unduly Reluctant to let others into own job
Specialist	Single-minded, self-starting, dedicated Provides knowledge and skills in rare supply	Contributes on only a limited front Dwells on specialised personal interests

are likely to be optional, such as certain seminars within your department. Within most educational institutions and hospitals it would be possible to spend many hours per week sitting in meetings, including research seminars, clinical review meetings, X-ray meetings, journal clubs, audit updates...

the list could go on. If you attended every possible meeting that could be construed as remotely relevant to your research project, you run the risk of not doing any other work! Clearly, you need to be selective and ask advice from your supervisor about what you should attend. You also need to think ahead and prepare for meetings, so that you gain the most benefit from them.

Supervisory meetings

When you meet with your supervisor, you should keep a written (or electronic) record of the matters discussed, action points and timescales for completing any agreed tasks. Arranging the date of the subsequent meeting is also helpful in preventing the project from drifting. If you keep summaries of these meetings electronically, they can also be sent by e-mail to your supervisor. Alternatively, many institutions now set up formats for you to keep an electronic portfolio, where you can store such documents but make them available to others where necessary and you may agree to deposit the records of your meetings in such a location. When agreed tasks are written down, there can be no ambiguity about what was decided at any later date.

In addition to making a record of meetings, you should ensure that you are adequately prepared for each meeting with the supervisor. You may want to take the responsibility for preparing an agenda. Remember to take your laboratory book, but also any results you want to present for discussion, a list of any questions you may have and anything else relevant. For example, you may want to ask about a journal article you have come across. Take a hard copy of the article because one of you may need to refer to some aspect of the article. You should also think about the immediate next steps of your project, so that you are actively planning your own work and not just carrying out what your supervisor tells you to do.

Seminars, journal clubs and other meetings

These may be organised on a laboratory basis, if you are part of a large team, or at the departmental level. Usually one or more individuals have the responsibility for presenting information to an audience, who are then expected to participate by asking questions and making comments. You may be expected to take a turn and present your work to a wider audience than just your supervisor, in which case you will have a lot of preparatory work (see Chapter 6). Even when you are not the star turn, you should still regard meetings of this type as an occasion where you are an active participant and not an opportunity to sit quietly, either listening or cogitating on unrelated matters. The best way of maintaining engagement with what is being presented is to make written notes during the presentation because you are then obliged to maintain your concentration. In the unfortunate event that a seminar or presentation is of a poor standard, or you find yourself wondering what on earth the speaker is talking about (and we have all experienced that situation!) you can analyse exactly what is going wrong. One scenario is that the topic is not one that you are familiar with or the level at which it is being discussed is beyond what you have experienced. This can arise when the speaker is addressing the specialists and experts in the room, unaware of (or neglecting) others in a mixed audience. In this case, you could wait until the end and then ask either the speaker or another colleague if they would explain the main message for you in simple terms. If the topic is one with which you are familiar, but the standard of presentation is less than adequate, take note of exactly why you are not learning. Is it because the speaker is going too fast and the slides are too busy for you to fully catch the messages? Is the talk poorly constructed so there seems to be little logical thread? If the speaker mumbles or speaks in a monotone, it can be very difficult to listen to what is being said. By paying attention to what makes for a poor presentation, you can avoid the pitfalls when it is your turn.

Questions and discussion are a vital part of seminars and related presentations. Without any questions, the interaction between the speaker and the audience is only in one direction. If you have engaged with what you have been listening to, you are likely to have some questions, or to want to know more detail about one aspect or another. Never be anxious about asking questions. Do not be inhibited by the presence of senior staff in the audience; your question is equally as important as the one from your head of department. Staff are always pleased when students participate in questions and discussion because it shows they are involved in the event and not merely sitting passively.

As a student, you may find yourself in an audience comprising mainly qualified staff and listening to a talk directed at them. The speaker may assume a level of knowledge in the audience that you do not have. In such a situation, you may need to ask for more information in order to benefit fully from what is being discussed. The person speaking at a seminar may not know that there are students in the audience. A courteous request along the lines of, 'Please could you say a little more about Bloggs' disease and its diagnosis, for the benefits of the students in the audience?' should provide you with the information you need. A good speaker will never mind being asked for more information because he or she will want all the audience to understand fully what is being said. Also, if there is something that you do not understand, it is likely that others in the room are in the same situation and will be pleased to have clarification. Never be embarrassed to ask a simple question; remember that 'the only stupid question is the one you were afraid to ask'.

Finally, at the conclusion of a seminar or presentation, make a brief summary in your laboratory book of the key learning points and, in particular, anything you may want to take forward to enhance your own project. This could include getting a copy of a specific manuscript or discussing a particular point in depth with your supervisor. You may not have such 'action points' after every talk you listen to, but with a few exceptions they should have enhanced your knowledge and understanding in ways you can identify.

SUMMARY

The working relationship between a supervisor and a student should be synergistic, with both individuals contributing equally but differently. Aim to build a professional, but friendly relationship.

You are likely to be part of a team. Think about how the team operates and how individual members interact. Make reasonable allowances for the shortcomings of others and think about how your own behaviour affects the team.

Over the course of your project, you will have different meetings with your supervisor and others. Make the most of these opportunities by having an agenda (if the meeting relates to your project) and by keeping notes of what has been learned or decided.

Further reading

http://www.studyskills.soton.ac.uk/research_skills/Research_Topic/crt_05.htm   (last accessed 14 January 2013).

Chapter 4 **Making progress**

CHAPTER OVERVIEW

This chapter highlights the importance of continually reviewing the data collected and keeping abreast of analysis to ensure as far as is possible that unforeseen errors do not arise. Suggestions for coding data are given, and the security of data storage and backup is discussed. Deciding when to stop collecting data, to allow sufficient time for analysis and writing up, is important. The chapter discusses how to decide when data collection should be completed.

This chapter could aptly be called 'keeping your nose to the grindstone', since it refers to applying yourself conscientiously to your work during the main data collection period of your project. Each project will be different, but many will have times when the data collection becomes tedious. This is when you must guard against falling into the trap of losing interest or commitment and be continually looking critically at your data.

Reviewing your progress during data collection

Provided that you prepared a detailed project plan, possibly along the lines of Figure 2.1, you should be working to a schedule that ensures the project is completed by the due date without the later stages being compressed. Figure 2.1 shows that several strands of the project run in parallel, so that on any given day the student might be doing one of two or three different tasks – each of which might be subdivided into smaller tasks. Your ability to manage your time and prioritise your work is likely to be more important in your

How to do your Research Project: A Guide for Students in Medicine and the Health Sciences, First Edition. Caroline Beardsmore.
© 2013 John Wiley & Sons, Ltd. Published 2013 by John Wiley & Sons, Ltd.

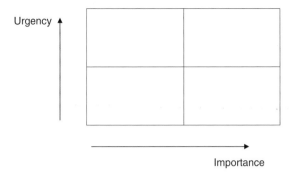

Figure 4.1 Matrix of importance and urgency.

research project than in other parts of your course, since you generally have more freedom and, therefore, more responsibility to get things done. While your project planner shows what you expect to be doing over the weeks and months of the project, it does not indicate what you expect to be doing on any given day. In planning your work, some things may be on fixed days and times (e.g. outpatient clinics, supervision meetings, departmental seminars). How you prioritise the other things can make all the difference to how smoothly your project proceeds. You may be familiar with the concept where tasks can be placed in a matrix of importance and urgency as illustrated in Figure 4.1.

Rather than jotting down a list of the tasks you need to complete, try positioning them in the matrix where it will be obvious that things in the upper right quadrant should take priority over the others.

The urgency/importance matrix is useful but you will probably find that you can only be effective at some of your tasks for limited periods of time before you need a break. An example might be data entry that is mind-numbingly boring but, more particularly, prone to an increasing number of errors with longer periods of time spent on the task. Extended time spent at a microscope or computer screen can lead to eye strain or headaches and is not a good idea. In contrast, many people find they can write more effectively when they have a long block (say 3–4 hours) of uninterrupted time. Draw up your work timetable to take account of such factors. When you are faced with new or unfamiliar tasks, do not leave them until the end of a day or week in case they take more time than you imagined or you find that you have to seek help or advice. Finally, do not overlook your own natural tendency to be more alert at certain times of the day than others; do not waste times of maximum effectiveness on tasks that do not merit it!

Sometimes the data collection parts of the project place particular demands on the student. It might be that the participants in your study are only prepared to take part in the evenings or at weekends. If you have a patient-based project that requires you to be available whenever particular patients are admitted, you may need to sacrifice some of your evening or weekends. If you are doing a laboratory project, you might find that some of your experiments run far longer than others and you may be required to continue working much later than you anticipated. You may have to share access to certain pieces of equipment with other people, so that you might have to start early in the mornings or work late in order to get the time that you need. Many research scientists make personal sacrifices of one sort or another in order that their work flourishes, and you should expect to do the same. Provided that you maintain a reasonable work–life balance and are not neglecting your health or other responsibilities, this should not be seen as a problem, but rather as part and parcel of a successful research career. Such personal sacrifices are not restricted to research or to medical or health-related professions.

Reviewing your data

In some research, the outcome cannot be known or predicted until all the data have been collected. This would be the case with a double-blind trial when the 'unblinding' takes place at the end. In some cases, you may get an overall impression of the likely results as the work proceeds. In other cases, you might be collecting the data but not be able to predict the final outcome. A preliminary or interim analysis can be helpful part-way through the data collection phase of a project to show whether sufficient data have been collected to achieve the project aims. Such a preliminary analysis can be useful because you can begin to prepare the Results and Discussion sections of your Dissertation, provided that you accept the chance that outcomes could change when data collection is complete. Some students might be tempted to run a preliminary analysis virtually every time they add a new set of results, whereas others may focus on getting their data and deliberately avoid looking at what it might show. An approach midway between these extremes is best.

You should always be alert to the quality and the technical acceptability of the data. Some projects involve taking recordings or measurements that only later get analysed, perhaps using a specific computer program or a piece of equipment. It may be the case that some samples are processed in batches, usually because the time or expense of setting up and calibrating equipment for the process is such that it is only worthwhile for several samples at a time. If you have mistakes or flaws in the way you collect your data or samples, you run the risk of much of the data being unreliable and/or unusable. Your project might involve collecting respiratory signals such as exhaled carbon dioxide and tidal volume. If the volume-measuring device is inserted the wrong way into the mouthpiece, the volume signal will be inverted on the monitor. This is not obvious on casual inspection because the subject is clearly breathing in and out, but if you look carefully at the recordings you should detect your error before you have wasted time and possibly lost data. When writing down results or readings, think whether what you are recording is realistic for the subject. When working with human subjects, height and weight are frequently and easily measured, but errors can – and do – occur. An example from my own experience happened when a laboratory cleaner altered the settings on the scales so that the digital reading appeared as pounds instead of kilograms. Although this gave gross errors it was not recognised immediately. It is not difficult to find people of average height (175 cm) who weigh 50 kg and others who weigh 110 kg, so unless the person reviewing the body weight had seen and remembered the subjects the data could be lost.

A good system of keeping records can help you to pick up on unexpected changes that alert you to possible errors. You may well find that equipment that is calibrated regularly has a calibration log book associated with it, so that it is a simple matter to look back and pinpoint a date when any sudden change occurred. If you are the person who observes a major change in calibration, or finds that a piece of equipment throws up an error message or does not seem to be functioning in the usual manner, do not ignore this even though it might continue to provide an output. The output may be unreliable or it might be a sign of impending failure. You may be able to do some 'troubleshooting' yourself in the first instance, or ask for help to sort out the problem.

In addition to reviewing data for quality and acceptability, think about the implications of your findings as your project progresses. Are you getting results that will fulfil the aims of your project? For example, you might be measuring a particular metabolite in urine, expecting to find a wide range of concentrations from different subjects. If you find that virtually all your subjects have a reading that is below the detection limits of your assay, you are not going to be able to say much when you write your dissertation. Knowing the problem in the early stages allows you to check your protocol, and then to make some decisions, such as trying a different assay, or focusing on a different metabolite.

By reviewing your data as it is collected you may find that it suggests new ideas that you might be able to explore. Do not automatically dismiss chance observations; simply noticing that newborn infants with jaundice did better when nursed on the sunny side of the nursery led to the introduction of pho-totherapy for the condition and a huge reduction in the need for exchange transfusions. In addition to any overall patterns in your results, look for outliers in your data – measurements that deviate markedly from the norm. Sometimes these are the consequence of an error on your part that can be corrected; on other occasions you may find an explanation that leads to the data being discounted. You might be making 24-hour recordings of variation in body temperature and find that one individual appeared to have a particularly high temperature. If he developed influenza the day following your recording you would not include his data as coming from healthy volunteers. You might, however, include it as an illustration of temperature changes at the onset of illness to contrast with data from your healthy group. Make sure you keep all your data; this is mandatory for studies involving human subjects and good laboratory practice in all other situations.

Data storage and security

There are several reasons for keeping data and therefore there may be more than one location where it is to be found. Clinical data pertaining to patients should be placed in their notes and the Case Report Form/Case Record Form (CRF) and stored securely. Sometimes data are also retained in laboratory records. Depending on the nature of your project, it is likely that you will also have data in your laboratory book and very possibly stored on a computer as well. You should be familiar with the principles of data protection (which have been enshrined in law for several years). Any breaching of the law could result in the halting of your research – and likely that of others in your laboratory or workplace setting, so do not take risks with data. Develop (or adapt) a system of labelling your samples or numbering your subjects that prevents you from transgressing the Data Protection Act. Information could be included in your coding system that helped you organise data on a spreadsheet without revealing personal information. Imagine that you had measurements from healthy controls and patients who were involved in a randomised controlled trial. Furthermore, you wanted to clearly differentiate males and females and know the date of testing. You might have a 10-digit/character identifier as follows:

Digit 1: 0 for control, 1 for a patient

Digit 2: 0 for control, A for active treatment, P for placebo (*NB* it is often useful to be able to distinguish controls from all patients combined; hence the use of two distinguishing characters)

Digit 3: M or F to signify gender

Digits 4–7: date and month of testing

Digits 8–10: subject number

If you saw the identifiers 00F1701003 and 1AF1901007, you would know that the first was a female control subject tested on 17 January and the third in your study group, and that the second was a female patient who was on active treatment tested on 19 January and the seventh in the study group.

Having decided on an identifying system, you can then proceed to collect and store data in whatever method is most appropriate. In some cases this will be your laboratory book if the amount of data is modest. If this is the case, you should seriously consider scanning in pages from the laboratory book with the essential results because loss or damage to the book would be disastrous. In many other cases you will want to use a database or a spreadsheet that you will update manually when data are acquired. While this may seem straightforward, it is well worth planning with care, especially if you have more than one set of measurements for each subject or experiment. You might see some subjects once only but others on two or three occasions. Should you organise a spreadsheet with strictly one row of data per subject, extending across many columns for the repeat visits? Or should you have one row per visit? Perhaps each subject merits a separate worksheet in a workbook? Your decision on the best layout should be based on what is going to make the analysis easiest to perform, and for this you may want to seek statistical advice. Data can be reorganised, copied and pasted but each time this is done there is the risk of error, and time is taken up that could be used for other things. Devote some time to finding the best format and stick to it.

If your data are to be stored electronically, your institutional computing service would almost certainly provide a daily backup that is much more secure than a laptop and memory stick, both of which can be lost or stolen. Use a system of identifying data files with the date of creation or update, so you are always working with the most recent version, but retain the penultimate version unopened in case of a major computer failure and the loss of information when you have your master file open.

If your data collection is going well you may be tempted to collect as much as possible, but you must leave sufficient time for analysis and completion of your write-up. One of the things that will require good judgement is when to stop collecting data.

How much data do you need? How do you know when to stop?

In many cases this is almost impossible to answer. The amount of data you are likely to collect will depend on the nature of your project and the time available to you. Your project might be a library project, reviewing the evidence about a particular topic such as the effects of fluoride in drinking water on dental health. At the outset, you could easily be overwhelmed at the sheer number of publications on the topic, so that you hardly knew where to start, let alone stop! Once you have worked out how to be selective in your reading, you may find that the information available is still more than you could possibly cover, and you will need to decide when 'enough is enough'. This may involve deciding what aspects of the topic are **not** going to feature in the review and how far back into the historical literature you want to go. Early publications on many topics can be fascinating, but that is not a universal truth. Not all of them are relevant and they are less likely to be readily available than more modern papers. If you find that several key publications reference an early work then it is likely to be a seminal paper and important to get hold of, but unless a thorough historical review is a big part of your project, your time may be better spent on more recent publications. When reviewing an old paper, try to establish if the data are accurate or if the experimental techniques have been superseded. It may be that the data are robust, but the contemporaneous interpretation may be questionable in the light of later developments.

Medical and scientific journals are not all the same and some are much more prestigious than others. The prestige of a journal is usually expressed in terms of its Impact Factor, a numerical value based on the number of times the papers it publishes are cited in other papers. The journals with the highest impact factors will accept a smaller proportion of papers submitted for publication and therefore are usually considered better quality. If you have to make choices in what you cover, pay attention to the impact factors of the journals you are looking at. This is, of course, a generalisation and you should remember that a journal dedicated to a topic of interest to a small number of specialists will never have the impact factor of a journal such as *The New England Journal of Medicine* or *The Lancet*, which cover a broader range of topics.

The amount of data required for laboratory projects may not necessarily be dictated by statistical requirements: if your task is to develop a test to detect a given compound in urine, for example, you may not be required to refine it once the main method has been established. If time permits, however, you would probably want to extend the project to produce a quantitative assay, and some statistical techniques (e.g. regression analysis) would be required for this.

In quantitative research, however, it may be possible to perform power calculations in order to work out how many subjects or measurements to include in your study (the sample size) to obtain a meaningful result. The formulae for performing power calculations are available from textbooks of statistics but there is no substitute for securing statistical advice at the outset. Your supervisor may have already determined the extent of your experimental work, or there may be someone appointed to advise students on statistics. Some of the factors that are relevant to working out 'how much data is enough' are elaborated below. Once you have an appreciation of why they may be important you will be better placed to judge an appropriate point to stop your data collection.

Power calculations

In performing power calculations, you will need to know the variability of the measurements you plan to make and you will make certain assumptions or judgements about what you consider significant. Suppose your research question relates to nicotine and calorie intake. Let us assume that you are testing the hypothesis that mice given nicotine consume less feed than control mice. Your experimental protocol involves two groups of mice of the same strain, age, sex and bodyweight (to within a few grams). They are allowed access to unlimited feed and water. You plan to give the experimental animals regular injections of nicotine and the controls will have sham (or dummy) injections. You will know how much feed they consume by weighing the feeders each day. What you need to think about is over what period of time the experiments will run and how many mice you will include. If you did not do any preparatory calculations, you might start off with five mice in each of the two groups (one experimental, one control) and record the daily food consumption. You could record your data in a table (Table 4.1), calculating the mean consumption for each group.

The mean food consumption in the treated group is less than that of the controls, but a casual glance of the data shows that there is a lot of overlap between the two groups. This is more clearly observed in an illustration than a table (Figure 4.2). The mean difference is small and most people would accept that it might have arisen by chance. The hypothesis has not been satisfactorily tested because the data are not sufficient to answer the question.

You would probably agree that if you repeated the same experiment, but this time you used 500 mice in each group instead of 5, and found the same difference in food consumption (5.5 g vs. 5.0 g), then you would be more certain that you were looking at a meaningful finding. You would have made 1000 measurements of food consumption instead of just 10, and would

Table 4.1 Daily food consumption of control mice and those treated with nicotine

Mouse number	Daily food consumption (g)	
	Control	**Nicotine**
1	5.5	6.0
2	4.5	3.5
3	6.0	5.0
4	6.5	5.0
5	5.5	5.5
Mean	5.6	5.0

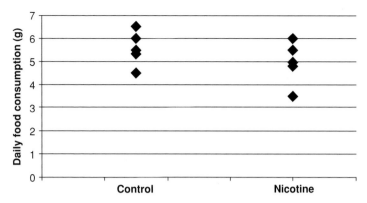

Figure 4.2 Daily food consumption of control mice and those treated with nicotine.

feel more secure in the results of your experiment. An alternative tactic would be to retain the services of the same original 10 mice but continue to weigh their feeders on a daily basis until you have accumulated 1000 measurements by that approach. This is less satisfactory because if you have one mouse whose food consumption is extreme, your results may be more skewed than if you used 500 mice. Either way, any demonstrated effect of nicotine on food consumption would be more convincing if backed up with many more measurements. This, however, brings with it other considerations, since purchasing and housing laboratory animals is very costly. If you are required to inject each mouse on a daily basis and weigh their feeders, this will take a huge amount of time. Aside from this, there are ethical constraints because it is unethical to subject the mice to injections unnecessarily. What you really need to work out in advance is how many mice you need to study, and over what period of time, to be secure in your conclusions.

You should consider what difference in food consumption, exactly, would be significant. The example above suggests that there could be a drop in food consumption of 10% in the treated mice. This would seem reasonably important – after all, we would probably notice an effect on both hunger and body weight if we reduced our calorie intake by 10% over more than a couple of days. But what if the average drop in food consumption was only 0.05 g per day? Apart from the difficulty of measuring such a small change, would it be important? In approaching a research question of a quantitative nature, you will need to make some judgements based on scientific knowledge and common sense.

One of the contributing factors to the inconclusive outcome shown above is that the food consumption varies between different mice. This is known as between-subject variation. Based on the data shown above, you have no idea whether each mouse has exactly the same food consumption every day or whether there is within-subject variation to be taken into account. Where there is less variation in the data you are collecting, fewer subjects are required to demonstrate a difference between groups. The variability in a measurement is usually expressed as a standard deviation (SD), shown alongside the mean. Thus you might find the information above written along the lines of 'the mean (SD) food consumption of the mice was 5.2 (± 0.85) g per day'.

Knowledge of the variability of the measurement you are making and a judgement about what you consider a significant change are important in working out the sample size you require. The final consideration is the power of the study to detect a significant difference between groups, if one exists. It gives a guide to the certainty of the conclusions. The power is usually expressed as a percentage, typically 80% or 90% power. The more measurements or subjects you include, the more powerful the study. In contrast, if you do not include sufficient subjects your study may not show a significant outcome when (in reality) it exists, simply because it was underpowered.

In many situations the variability of your measurements may be known, so by setting what you consider to be a significant effect and the power of the study, it is a simple matter to work out the sample size required.

The importance of statistical analysis

In the example above, a power calculation would be straightforward provided that we knew the variability of the food consumption of the mice. One aspect of many research projects is working with data that, because of their very nature, provide more of a challenge. This is where advice from someone who has statistical knowledge is invaluable, and if you also understand some basic statistical considerations you can avoid some of the commoner mistakes made by the unwary. If you are discussing data analysis with a statistician, he or she is likely to be more interested in how the data are collected and presented rather than your field of study. Of course, anyone with whom you discuss the statistical aspects of your project will want to know what the project is all about, but they will be thinking about the data and analysis more than the topic. Try to see things from their perspective by considering these two possible questions:

Are verrucas commoner in people who attend public swimming pools on a frequent basis than in those who never swim?

Is an allergy to horses commoner in people who work with horses (grooms, jockeys, livery staff) than those who do not?

The statistical approach to answering these questions is likely to be identical, even though the consequences of getting a verruca cannot be compared with developing an allergy.

Some of the key points that a statistician will want to know about when considering the approach to analysis are outlined below:

- **Data that are not normally distributed about the mean.** A normal distribution refers to data that are equally scattered above and below the mean. An example would be height – you might read that the mean height for men is 176.8 cm with a standard deviation of 5.8 cm. Any man has an equal chance of being taller or shorter than the mean. In contrast, the number of children born to women cannot be normally distributed. The mean number of children born to European women might be 2.3, but a moment's consideration would bring to mind that while some women will have no children, others will have many more. You can also appreciate that expressing the average number of children born to women as a mean value is not necessarily the best way, and reporting the commonest value (or mode) may be more sensible.

- **Continuous or categorical data.** Height measurement is an example of a continuous measurement; theoretically, you could measure height to any number of decimal places. Examples of categorical data include numbers of children, gender or marital status. Individuals can fall into only one category. Categorical data can also include that which has been created or defined by the researcher. You might ask your participants about their diet and divide them into the following four categories: (i) omnivores, (ii) people who eat fish but are otherwise vegetarian, (iii) vegetarians and (iv) vegans. With this type of information, you have the possibility of combining two categories (you may find that you have so few vegans that you want to combine them with the vegetarians). Some categories may have an element of increase (e.g. disease categorised into mild, moderate, severe, or age divided into <20, 20–24, 40–60, >60 years) whereas others such as gender do not.

- **Missing data.** Missing data can arise for many reasons, particularly when working with human subjects. If each subject is required to do several things, one or more might be missing. A subject may choose not to answer a question in a questionnaire, or be unable to complete a particular component of a project. You might find that one piece of equipment breaks down part-way through a test and the data are lost. Sometimes this is not a major issue and the data can be presented with a note of how many measurements were included for each aspect of the project. In other situations, the missing data may come predominantly from one group and could potentially bias the data.

- **Dropout rate.** If you are making repeated measurements over time, some of your subjects may withdraw part-way through the usual period of inclusion. This can reduce the significance of your results but, if you anticipate the number of subjects likely to withdraw, you might recruit extra subjects at the outset to increase the chance of a sufficient number completing.
- **Sources of bias and generalising your findings.** Bias happens when your results are skewed to reflect one group in preference to another, and can lead to incorrect conclusions. If your data are from a defined source, your conclusions are relevant for that source and you may not generalise to other groups. Sometimes this is well recognised; for example drug metabolism can be influenced by age and data from young, healthy adults cannot be presumed to reflect what happens in children or the elderly. Information derived from one species may not apply to others (Prof Brown's project on gastric motility, mentioned in Chapter 1, might **suggest** things relevant for humans but cannot be taken as proof). In other cases you will need to think possible sources of bias and how they might arise. Socioeconomic status affects many aspects of human health but it can be difficult to avoid as a source of bias. For example, participants in a research study are likely to have their expenses reimbursed but the poorest members of our society may worry about how long this might take. They may be discouraged from joining a study that required attendance at a hospital or university if they could not be certain that their travel expenses or car park charge was not going to be reimbursed in cash on the day of participation.
- **Confounders.** Confounders are things that, if not taken into account, can bias or confuse a study. An example would be the association between smoking, breastfeeding and socioeconomic status. If your project looked at an aspect of child health in relation to breastfeeding, you might reach an incorrect conclusion. Your findings may instead relate to the exposure of children to cigarette smoke, since there is a strong link between maternal smoking and the lack of breastfeeding. Alternatively, your results may relate to socioeconomic status, since both breastfeeding and smoking are closely related to this.

The list of statistical considerations is not exhaustive but should start you thinking about how best to analyse your results. Remember also that the amount of data that can be collected in the time available for your project may be limited, so that your analysis may be restricted to one key outcome. You may not have enough information to be able to answer more detailed questions. If you have an understanding of potential statistical pitfalls and limitations you can, however, address this in the Discussion section of your dissertation.

Beginning your data analysis

There may be a small number of projects where any statistical analysis cannot begin until the data collection is complete, perhaps, because certain types of samples are processed as a batch and are not available until the end. In many cases, it is possible to perform a preliminary analysis once some of the data are available. There are several advantages to doing an interim analysis. You will have the experience of actually doing the data analysis and interpreting the outcomes, you can begin to think about the most effective ways of displaying your data, you may get a strong hint about what the final outcomes are likely to be and you may be alerted to a possible unforeseen difficulty that you may be able to rectify while you still have the time to do so. Reviewing your data during the course of the project may prompt new ideas or questions. Statistical analysis of data is almost always done using a statistical analysis package or application on your computer, of which there are many. If your data are on an Excel^{TM} spreadsheet you may use the statistical function that accompanies this, or there are other packages that are likely to be available through your institutional IT services. Two of the commonest are the Statistical Package for the Social Sciences (SPSS) and Stata (name derived from statistics and data). While none of these are difficult to use, you will need to invest time in familiarising yourself with how to use them (those online tutorials are there for a purpose!) and seek advice on which is likely to be the best for your purposes. People will have their individual preferences, based on things like the appearance and the functionality of the associated graphical displays.

Having acquired a basic familiarity with a statistical package, you can begin to analyse your data and possibly draw some tentative conclusions. This is always an exciting stage of any research, when things seem to come together at last. It can be very tempting to perform a reanalysis with every new test added to your database, perhaps in the hope that something of statistical significance will emerge, but this is best avoided since it will take up time that is better spent on other things. Do present your preliminary observations to your supervisor and others in the team so that you can benefit from their ideas and experience.

If your research project is qualitative your data analysis will use a different approach, since you will be interested in developing hypotheses or ideas, or identifying themes, perhaps emerging from interviews or focus groups. The analysis can parallel the data collection, rather than be sequential to it. At the outset of the project you may be overwhelmed by the sheer volume of information you collect, whether this is in electronic format (such as the recordings of interviews that subsequently get transcribed) or your own text. The organisation of the information, development of a systematic interrogation of the material and the reflection required for valid conclusions to be drawn, need to start early and be continuous. For many students, the concepts involved in qualitative research will be novel and you will need time to grasp and apply them alongside the information-gathering processes. In contrast to most quantitative research, where the final outcomes may suddenly become available at the conclusion of statistical analysis, qualitative outcomes emerge more gradually and the process of refining your analysis can be protracted. Start early.

Practical considerations that might limit your project

An important part of project planning is not simply performing a power calculation, but working out the feasibility of what can be done with the time and resources available. In cases where power calculations cannot be performed (perhaps because the variability of a measurement is unknown), the number of measurements made might be worked out on a purely pragmatic basis. It can sometimes be difficult to predict how much data can be collected in a given period of time and unpredictable events can upset even the best-planned project. We can review some new examples and those from previous chapters and consider what might dictate the extent of data collection, and identify some data-related or statistical considerations for each one:

Joe's project involved using a questionnaire about diet to see whether medical and nursing students had a healthier diet than other students.

Without proper planning, he could run the risk of collecting a lot of data without knowing how to analyse it. Questionnaire-based studies may appear conceptually simple but can be fraught with difficulties. Sometimes it is possible to use questionnaires that have been published or validated, which means that other people have developed and used them and ironed out the problems. A classic example of this would be the International Study of Asthma and Allergies in Childhood (ISAAC) questionnaire, which is available in many languages and formats for children of different ages. While no questionnaire is perfect, anyone wanting to work in the area of paediatric asthma or allergy would be best advised to use ISAAC questions, rather than try to reinvent this particular wheel. Where no such validated questionnaire exists, then running a small pilot project with a trial questionnaire can be a useful means of identifying problems before too much work gets done. Joe's project might lend itself to this if he had sufficient time.

Joe's questionnaire included questions about the type of diet during childhood, proximity to shops and fast-food outlets, and cooking facilities available in the student accommodation, as well as food consumed over a week. Assuming that access to students was not going to limit his data collection, he could get hundreds of completed questionnaires to analyse. What Joe might not have thought about was the time he might need to enter all the data into his computer. If he had only 120 completed questionnaires, but it took him 10 minutes to enter the data for each one, then that would require 20 solid hours of data entry before the analysis could start. Data entry cannot be done without regular breaks and even the most careful person will make errors. Sometimes these become blindingly obvious (if Joe produced a frequency histogram of the portions of fruit eaten each day that showed one individual consumed 45 portions, the error would be obvious. In this case, it might be a typing error and the keys for 4 and 5 were accidently both struck simultaneously). Other errors are more difficult to detect, which is why some well-resourced studies use double data entry, and software to identify discrepancies between data sheets that should be identical.

The limiting factor for Joe might, therefore, be purely practical, that is, the time it would take him to collect the questionnaires and enter all the data. He could solve this problem by making his questionnaire available online, although his response rate might then be reduced. He could also cut down on the number of questions and the scope of his project. If a pilot study had shown that all the students lived in accommodation with access to a full range of cooking facilities, then it is unlikely that he would be able to say anything novel about this, and it might be best to drop questions about cooking facilities completely.

In terms of analysis, Joe would have to consider how to decide whether the diet of one group of students was healthier than another. He might decide to use a combination of (i) the number of portions of fruits and vegetables consumed each day, (ii) the number of times the student ate from a 'fast food' outlet per week and (iii) whether or not the student consumed more alcohol than the recommended guidelines of 2–3 units per day for women or 3–4 units per day for men. What might complicate his analysis, however, is a possible association between drinking alcohol and consuming takeaways and fast food. Statistical techniques can take account of such associations if there is sufficient data, but this might be beyond the scope of a student project. Joe's analysis might be restricted to basic statistics, but an appreciation of what might be done with more data and the limitations of his analysis, should feature in the Discussion section of his dissertation.

Hannah's project focused on the different types of pain relief used in childbirth. It was mainly a library project but included a review of the records over a 3-month period from the delivery suite of the hospital where she was based.

Hannah would need to decide how to divide her time between the two aspects of her project. If she worked on the two aspects in parallel she might find that each part enhanced her approach to the other, so that her reading might help her decide what aspects of the hospital notes she would want to review, and examining the notes could suggest things she might research in the literature. Furthermore, a parallel approach might help her to balance the work so that the final dissertation did not overemphasise one aspect at the cost of the other. The library or analytical part of any project could be never-ending, so that deciding early on about the scope of the reading and the plan of the dissertation would be essential to achieving balance in the dissertation. The issues surrounding the 3-month review of records would be different. The approximate number of records for review would be known in advance, but Hannah would need to establish how long it would take her to access and review each one. As with Joe's project, she would need to decide in advance what information she wanted to collect and how it might be analysed. She might limit her review to describing the types of pain relief used in the hospital, and whether the frequency of use was different according to the obstetric history of the mother and/or which health professional attended the delivery, or she could collect more information and include a more detailed statistical analysis. Her supervisor should provide guidance on the amount of information and analysis she should expect to handle in the course of the project, allowing for sufficient time to write a good dissertation.

Emma's project was designed to measure the density of a certain receptor on cells from the airway smooth muscle of experimental mice. There were three groups of mice; two were pretreated with different agents and the third were controls.

Since this project uses experimental animals, the amount of data Emma could collect would be limited by the number of mice in the study. Knowing that the technique for assessing receptor density was complex and required several stages, it would be sensible for Emma to become experienced at every stage of the work before pressing too far ahead with using her experimental animals. It could be disastrous if she took all her samples to the penultimate stage of the procedure, only to find that she could not perform the last step because she had overlooked something at the start. Once she is competent at all aspects of the practical procedures, Emma should be able to schedule all her experimental work within the time available to her. Unlike some of the other projects, those involving animals are rarely open-ended. Although Emma might be able to schedule some of the work purely at her own convenience (e.g. histology and counting receptors), the animal work might be dependent on the availability of laboratory facilities or other people. She should plan ahead to ensure that her project is not curtailed by things that could have been avoided.

Projects from Chapter 1
Melanie had the choice of two projects:

- Dr Black's project was based in a maternity hospital and the aim was to compare the levels of progesterone in the serum of women at different stages of pregnancy. The role of the student was to collect the blood samples after the medical research fellow had taken written consent, take them to the laboratory for analysis, enter the results into the computer and relate them to questionnaire data that had been collected by the research midwife (provided that she had been available at the time of the relevant clinic visit).

Melanie is dependent on the medical research fellow and the midwife to secure written consent and questionnaire data. Assuming that there is no shortage of women attending the maternity hospital, the final number of women in Melanie's study will be limited by the motivation and availability of other people. Accident or illness or move to alternative employment could jeopardise the project. Melanie would want to know how variable the measurement of progesterone was and whether this altered during pregnancy.

- Dr Green's project was designed to look for tumour markers for bowel cancer on previously collected preserved specimens. The specimens were all available and the protocol for preparing and staining the slides, and detecting the tumour markers, was already established. The associated clinical data had been collected and was available on a computer spreadsheet.

The specimens were collected in advance of the project so the final number of samples is known in advance. What is not known at the outset is which markers are expressed on the specimens and how they relate to clinical data (this is the focus of the research!). If Melanie is fortunate she will find some clear associations between certain markers and clinical data. If her results are borderline she may be in a position to calculate the size of a study required to provide clear-cut answers. In terms of the amount of data available for the project report, this would be the safer option.

Philip also had the choice of two projects:

- Dr White's project was based in a busy general practice and focused on finding out why patients sought medical advice or intervention following day-case surgery. The project included patient interviews, including assessment of their levels of satisfaction and reviews of hospital case notes.

Several factors could limit the number of interviews Philip might complete, beginning with the number of patients in the practice who underwent day-case surgery. Arrangements for interview could be important, since fewer patients might agree to attend the GP practice than would be happy to participate if Philip went to their home. If it was a rural practice, Philip might need his own transport to visit patients over a wide area. When it comes to reviewing hospital case notes, Philip might not be able to trace these very easily, since it is not unknown for notes to go missing. The nature of this project means that the results are likely to be descriptive, although the assessment of level of satisfaction could be quantitative or semi-quantitative. This could be a great project if Philip was resourceful and highly committed, but a student who expected the data to be handed to them 'on a plate' would do less well.

- Professor Brown's project was laboratory based and looked at gastric motility in a guinea pig model. Philip would need to have an animal licence and would have a lot of 'hands-on' laboratory experience but no patient contact or overt clinical application.

Since this project involves work with experimental animals a Home Office licence would be required and the number of guinea pigs that could be used would be set out at the start. The number to be used would be the minimum compatible with achieving the scientific objectives. Philip would need to work carefully and to a strict protocol to minimise the variability in measurements of gastric motility, so that any changes induced by experimental interventions would be as clear as possible. The opportunity to repeat experiments on additional animals would be non-existent or very unlikely. A physiological preparation (in this case part of the intestinal tract in an organ bath) might be viable for several hours, enabling Philip to carry out repeated experiments, although this might require him to be in the laboratory until late into the evening.

Justifying the end point of a project

By now you will have realised that research is open-ended and that you could probably keep working well beyond normal retirement age! If you are fortunate you will have the sort of project where the amount of experimental work or data collection was known in advance and you have achieved the target. For many students their project is curtailed in other ways and you should be clear about what limited the amount of work you covered, so that you can discuss it with your examiners, for example. In some cases you may have spent a lot of time and effort establishing a method before it became useful, or had unforeseen obstacles to your data collection. Without making this appear as a litany of excuses, make sure that this aspect of your work is included in your assessment so you can be given due credit. Beyond this, think about what you would have done if you had more time/patients/resources available to you, so that you can demonstrate that you have the vision to take the project to the next stage should circumstances permit.

SUMMARY

Even during those times when your project is running well and you may be
extremely busy collecting data, you should review your data for technical
acceptability at intervals. Unless there is good reason to delay, try not to
let data analysis build up in case there are unforeseen errors that could
invalidate the data.

Make sure that your information is stored securely and in compliance with any
pertinent regulations. Backup is essential.

Recognise that you may need to make personal sacrifices in the course of your
project. Research is rarely a '9 to 5' occupation.

Know when to stop data collection, whether this decision is based on evalua-
tion of statistical power or practical reasons.

Further reading

Greenhalgh, T. (2010) *How to Read a Paper: The Basics of Evidence-Based Medicine*,
4th edn, Wiley-Blackwell.

Bland, M. (2000) *An Introduction to Medical Statistics*, 3rd edn, Oxford Medical
Publications.

Chapter 5 **Writing up**

CHAPTER OVERVIEW

Writing up is often seen as the final part of the research project, but in reality it should happen alongside all other aspects. This chapter stresses the importance of becoming familiar with institutional guidelines at the outset and of making an early start to the writing-up. Emphasis is placed on structuring the dissertation that is an aid to planning. The precise structure can be adapted to the nature of the project; the clarity of the final product should be paramount. The dissertation can be enhanced by good illustrations and table layout. 'Writer's block' is common and the chapter suggests what to do when affected by this. Advice concerning the avoidance of plagiarism and revising the dissertation is provided.

Introduction

Your research project will count for nothing if it is not written up. You may have the sharpest intellect in your university, or be the most skilled student ever to work in a laboratory, but if you cannot write up your work in a satisfactory manner then nobody can learn from it or fully assess it. That would be a terrific waste of time, effort and energy by you and others you have worked alongside. If your research project has involved human volunteers or animal studies then the failure to disseminate the findings can be seen as unethical. If your project is to count for anything, it is imperative that your write-up is of the highest possible standard.

How to do your Research Project: A Guide for Students in Medicine and the Health Sciences,
First Edition. Caroline Beardsmore.
© 2013 John Wiley & Sons, Ltd. Published 2013 by John Wiley & Sons, Ltd.

Different institutions may refer to the written document by different names, such as a thesis, dissertation or project report. Since 'thesis' is the term usually used for a higher degree, the term 'dissertation' will be used in this book.

The dissertation is likely to be the longest piece of work you have written in your career and the prospect can appear daunting. This may be one reason why many students are tempted to put off writing until almost the last possible moment, only to find that it takes much more time than they originally thought. Many students procrastinate because they want to complete the practical work before beginning to write. The result is that the work submitted is not as good as it might have been, had the student allowed more time. Sometimes the early days of a project can be relatively quiet – the practical techniques need to be practised, the interlibrary loans are awaited, or the subject recruitment has not started. The savvy student will capitalise on this time not only by getting ahead with the reading and summarising the references but also by planning the dissertation.

The importance of starting early

It is never too early to begin work on the dissertation. 'Work on the dissertation' does not necessarily mean that you begin to write incomparable prose from the first moment your fingers touch the keyboard. Rather, it implies a degree of planning that underpins the subsequent stages of the production of the dissertation. The blank screen or sheet of white paper can induce a sinking feeling even in people who write extensively. Most of us can identify with the displacement activity that we indulge in to avoid the writing tasks. Suddenly it becomes very important to attend to a pressing domestic task or a social matter rather than face up to the task of writing. Try to avoid displacement activity – the consequences of **not** completing any given domestic task are usually trivial when compared with the importance of your dissertation.

The trick is to plan a detailed outline of the dissertation, and break it down into small components that can be tackled individually. The most straightforward way of doing this is to write the contents page first, with all the chapters, sections, subsections, sub-subsections and so on, so you can see the complete outline of the finished product (see 'Joe's project' below). This structure may get revised over the course of time but that does not matter. The contents pages will give you a scaffolding to start writing. Next you can decide if some written work you may already have done can be used, either in its entirety or after some modifications. For example, if you have written a Standard Operating Procedure (SOP) for something, it may fit into your Methods section. If you did an essay or report at an earlier stage in your studies, are there parts that can be used in the dissertation? Suddenly you discover that you have already started writing.

What form should the dissertation take?

Your university or department will provide information about the regulations relating to the dissertation. These may be lax (e.g. just giving a guide on the length or word count) or they may be much more detailed, indicating the width of margins, line spacing, font and font size, referencing style, number of figures allowed and so on. Familiarise yourself with the requirements at the outset. In most cases, you should be able to examine examples of dissertations from previous students and it is well worth looking at a selection of these. If you know the grade given for each dissertation, you will be able to gain a feel for what constitutes an outstanding piece of work. Do bear in mind that the overall mark for a student project may include, for example, a component awarded on the basis of practical skills or performance in a viva examination – find out what proportion of marks are given to the dissertation from your own institution.

Structuring the dissertation

You may think you know how you will structure your dissertation. It is a well-known pattern:
• Abstract
• Aims (sometimes placed within or after Background and Introduction)
• Background and Introduction
• Materials and Methods
• Results
• Discussion and Conclusions
• References
When you look at examples of completed dissertations, however, you will most probably find that they have been structured with a hierarchy of sub-headings. Some projects with different components may have several sections, each of which includes Methods and Results specific to that section. Working within the regulations of your institution, the key to structuring any piece of work lies in clarity. The reader needs to navigate his or her way around the dissertation, and the writer (you!) should make this as straightforward as possible by providing a sensible structure and clear signposting. Consider the examples below:

Joe's project involved using a questionnaire about diet to see whether medical and nursing students had a healthier diet than other students. Joe broke down his outline into various subsections, so he could have a clear vision at the outset of his final dissertation, before beginning any data collection

Abstract

Chapter 1. Background and Introduction

    1.1 Importance of diet, what constitutes a healthy diet

    1.2 Factors that might influence healthy diet

        1.2.1 Type of accommodation/cooking facilities

        1.2.2 Type of diet during upbringing, incl. ethnic foods

        1.2.3 Proximity to market/shops/fast food outlets

        1.2.4 Price of foodstuffs

        1.2.5 Importance of chosen foods for health/slimming etc.

    1.3 How to assess diet

        1.3.1 Food diaries

        1.3.2 Retrospective questionnaires

    1.4 Aim of project

Chapter 2. Methods

    2.1 Outline of study, ethics, permission

    2.2 Subject selection and recruitment

        2.2.1 Medical and nursing students

        2.2.2 Other students

    2.3 Questionnaire surveys

    2.4 Statistical methods

Chapter 3. Results

    3.1 Response rates, numbers in each group

    3.2 Comparison of diet

        3.2.1 Based on intake of (i) protein, (ii) fats, (iii) carbohydrate, (iv) vitamins and minerals

        3.2.2 Based on eating patterns (i) skipping breakfast, (ii) frequency of fresh fruit/veg, (iii) fast food, (iv) alcohol intake

    3.3 Differences between medics, nurses and other students

    3.4 (Possibly) Gender effects

Chapter 4. Discussion and Conclusions

    4.1 Main findings

    4.2 Limitations of the study

    4.3 Factors that might explain the results – quote some free text here

    4.4 Suggestions for future studies – and possible strategies that would improve diet of students

References

Appendix

Hannah's project focused on different types of pain relief used in childbirth. It was mainly a library project but included a review of the records over a 3-month period from the delivery suite of the hospital where she was based. She wanted a structure that linked these two aspects together, so she could draw conclusions relevant to her local patient population. At the beginning of her project, she drew up the following structure:

Chapter 1. Background and Introduction, aim of the project

    1.1 **Historical background** to pain relief in childbirth – including examples from different cultures

    1.2 **Different types of analgesic agents** – structure, mechanism of action, administration, indications and contraindications, possible side effects. Each agent considered in turn

One-page tabular summary of methods of pain relief commonly used in childbirth

    1.3 **Introduction to review of records**

Chapter 2. Methods employed with explanations and justifications (how were the delivery suite records accessed, which records were excluded (e.g. multiple births? women who went into labour but then required emergency caesarean section?), which data were recorded

Chapter 3. Results of review of records (frequency of use of different agents and factors associated with choice of pain relief, including maternal factors (first or subsequent delivery) and hospital related factors such as whether delivery attended by midwife or obstetrician)

    (Possibly some case studies to illustrate particular findings)

Chapter 4. Discussion, commenting on whether the local use of pain relief in childbirth was consistent with the best current recommendations. If not, what are the reasons why this might be so? Limitations of the review of records, such as possible sources of bias, generalisability of the findings. Suggestions for future studies

Chapter 5. Overarching conclusions

References

Appendices (including approval for the study, blank data collection forms, tabulated data (anonymised)

Emma's project was designed to measure the density of a certain receptor on cells from the airway smooth muscle of experimental mice. There were three groups of mice – two were pretreated with different agents and the third were controls. The technique for assessing the density of the receptor was complicated and required several stages. Although she initially tried writing her dissertation in the usual format, Emma found that the lengthy technical description of how to measure the receptor density disrupted the continuity of the dissertation by divorcing the main Methods from the Results. She eventually achieved a much clearer outcome by using the following structure:

Chapter 1. Background and Introduction, aim of the project

Chapter 2. Method of assessing receptor density, including how results are analysed and reported

Chapter 3. Main methods, including study design, equipment, all experimental procedures other than assessing receptor density, which was covered by the phrase 'receptor density was assessed as previously described'

Chapter 4. Results

Chapter 5. Discussion, which included a subsection on 'limitations of the methods'

Chapter 6. Conclusions and suggestions for further research

By encapsulating the section on assessing receptor density in a separate chapter, Emma's dissertation 'flowed' more smoothly and the reader had the option to read the dissertation without reference to this if he or she wanted to gain a simple overview.

What should each section contain?

The various sections of a dissertation serve different purposes and if the contents of one section are missing from the expected location or placed elsewhere the reader may struggle. It is not satisfactory to put everything down somewhere and hope that will suffice. While there may be different opinions about precisely where some items should be placed, there is a general consensus on the overall contents.

The **Title** may already be dictated by the project proposal set out by your supervisor and there may be a requirement to adhere to this. Sometimes the project completed by the student may not have developed as originally envisaged and the original title may be unsuitable. If you think you need to change the title, you should ask the course organiser if this is permissible. Other institutions may have a more relaxed approach and allow you to choose whatever title you want, perhaps with a limit on the number of words or characters. If you are deciding on a title for your own dissertation, you will want to give it some thought. It should convey something of the topic of your work and is best kept short. If you are tempted to think up a witty title, think very hard. A play on words that includes a clever reference to a contemporary film or album might be extremely tempting, but (a) the examiner may not recognise the reference and (b) it might seem very passé in a few years' time. Rambling titles that contain redundant words are generally less attention-grabbing than those that are more direct.

Consider the possible titles for the projects outlined above:

Joe's project:
'A Study to Investigate whether Medical and Nursing Students Eat More Healthily than Students of Other Disciplines'
   Versus 'The Student Diet: Is It Influenced by Degree Course?'

Hannah's project:
'A Report into Different Kinds of Pain Relief Used in Childbirth Including a Review of Options Used in Mytown General Hospital'
   Versus 'Pain Relief in Childbirth'

Emma's project
'Investigations into the Effect of Two Different Toxins on the Density of Thingummy Receptors on the Airway Smooth Muscle Cells of Mice'
   Versus 'Factors Influencing Thingummy Receptor Density in Airway Smooth Muscle'

You will want to strike a balance between something that is brief but punchy and a longer but perhaps more informative title. Try two or three versions and ask friends and colleagues which seems to work best.

In many institutions it is customary for the student to make an **acknowledgement** of help that he or she has received in working through their project. Such acknowledgements are typically placed at the front of the dissertation. If you have had direct financial support such as a bursary, then you will no doubt want to express your thanks at the outset. Unless something has gone very badly wrong with your supervision, you may wish to thank your supervisor, and any other person who has made an important contribution to your project. If you have worked with volunteers, either healthy people or patients, it is fitting to record your gratitude to them. There may be other individuals you want to mention, such as your parents or partner, and this is the place to do this.

The **Abstract** is almost always written last, but it will be read first and is likely to be the part that is read most. It is therefore absolutely vital to spend time writing a good abstract because it will function as the 'shop window' for your work. It is a brief overview of the complete study and is usually written with a restricted word count. You may be asked to write the abstract in a structured format, with a paragraph for Introduction, Methods, Results and Discussion, although this is not usual for a dissertation. It is, nonetheless, a good starting point. If your project has generated many results, you may need to include only the chief findings and leave the detailed sub-analyses for the main dissertation. You may be able to include a table within the abstract that would enable you to include more results, but check in advance if you want to do this. It is not usual to include any diagrams or illustrations in an abstract.

The **Aim** of the project needs to be clearly stated. Some people prefer this to be provided at the outset; others find it is better to provide the relevant background information before stating the precise aims or the research question.

The **Background and Introduction** will probably be written early. You may divide this section into its two component parts, or keep them united. The purpose of this section is to introduce your topic and to justify the work you have done yourself. Usually this section will conclude with a statement of the overall aims of your own work, so it is important that there is a build-up to this. One usual pattern is to begin with some 'broad brush' information about the scale of the medical problem that lies behind the project, then to focus on the particular aspect that underpins your research project. In writing this section of your dissertation, you will need to consider the balance between different sections and subsections. You may be tempted to try and include everything that is known about the topic but remember it is a dissertation, not a textbook. Using Emma's project (see above) as an example, she would probably include some information about the prevalence of asthma, mortality figures and healthcare costs, and the impact of the disease on individuals with asthma. She might move on to discuss the mechanisms of airway obstruction in asthma and the role of the airway smooth muscle. In the final parts of her Background and Introduction, she would write in some detail about the receptors on smooth muscle cells and the work in this defined area, leading in to the aim of her project with, if appropriate, a testable hypothesis. She would probably leave out anything to do with epidemiology, genetics or treatment of asthma since these aspects would be largely irrelevant to her project and use up too much of her limited word count.

Many students find that the first draft of the Background and Introduction turns out to be longer than they ultimately want it to be. Commonly, they will have referred to many previous studies that are relevant for their own work. Once the whole dissertation becomes more complete it may become obvious that some of the Background and Introduction is more relevant for the Discussion section and should be moved, resulting in a more balanced dissertation and better focus in the earlier part. Do not be too concerned if the first draft of the Background and Introduction exceeds your target word count (within reason!) as it is likely to be slimmed down at a later stage.

The **Methods** section can usually be written at an early stage. Whether you call this section Materials and Methods, or Equipment and Methods, or simply Methods, is a matter of what is appropriate for your project. The structure of this section will depend on the complexity of the piece of research, and on whether the techniques you are using are simple or require a lot of detailed description. Judicious use of hierarchical subheadings will help you organise this section, delineating the parts where you are describing how equipment is set up and calibrated from the other parts describing the study design. This is a section that generally benefits from flow charts and diagrams to show how your research question is being addressed. When describing your equipment, remember that the examiners may be unfamiliar with what you are doing, and a clear diagram, as in Figure 5.1, will be invaluable.

Figure 5.1 shows the precise circuitry used in the student's experimental work. A separate illustration (Figure 5.2) was also included in this student's

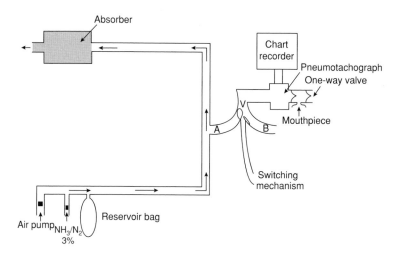

A: Ammonia + air limb   B: Room air limb   V: Balloon valve

Figure 5.1 Diagram of the equipment used to measure the sensitivity of upper airway reflexes. While this diagram does not give the reader any idea of what the equipment looked like in practice, it shows clearly the arrangements of different parts of the circuitry. (Courtesy of Dr Ben Prudon, reproduced with permission.)

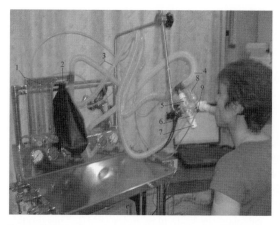

1. Air and ammonia flowmeters
2. 6 litre reservoir bag
3. Tubes carrying the ammonia/air mixture to the 2nd balloon valve
4. Tubes carrying the ammonia/air mixture to the absorber canister
5. 2nd Balloon valve
6. 1st Balloon valve
7. Entry point for room air in the 'air limb'
8. Exit point for exhaled air
9. Pneumotachograph connection

Figure 5.2 Equipment used to measure glottic reflex sensitivity. This figure shows the reader the appearance of the equipment used in Ben's project, with labels to indicate the component parts. (Courtesy of Dr Ben Prudon, reproduced with permission.)

dissertation. While it was not, perhaps, strictly necessary it provided a splash of colour and also conveyed an impression of what the experimental procedure was like at the time. Photographic records of work on progress are also useful if you are going to prepare a poster describing your work, so keep your camera handy! Even if your project is a library project or an audit, with little opportunity for an 'action shot', a colourful photograph on the cover or perhaps at the start of each chapter will add to the attractiveness of the dissertation. Returning to the three hypothetical student projects above, Joe could obviously illustrate his dissertation with pictures of different food types; Hannah's project might be illustrated with a photo of a heavily pregnant woman, and Emma might choose a colourful photomicrograph of the airway smooth muscle cells she was using. Do remember, however, that if you want to include photographs of people, especially patients, you should seek their written consent for this. If working with patients, the relevant NHS Trust will probably have a *pro forma* for recording consent to be photographed or videoed.

Some students will be using commercial equipment or techniques and will need to decide how much written detail to include in their Methods section. To some extent this will be governed by the overall word count, and sometimes references to published methods will suffice. You should know the basic principle behind each commercial method you employ, however, as accuracy and reliability might be influenced by the circumstances of your particular application. For example, if you understand that a pulse oximeter works by transmission and reception of light of particular wavelengths you will realise (i) that the oximeter probe you select should fit snugly on the subject's finger, without the chance of extraneous light impacting on the receptor and (ii) that transmitter and detector should be positioned opposite each other.

When the Methods section is complete, it should be sufficiently detailed for another person to duplicate your work should they want to do so. You should provide details of equipment manufacturers, sources of materials and all the necessary technical detail for the work to be repeated. Depending on the nature of your project, you may include a subsection headed 'Method of Analysis', which would describe what you did with the data after collection. This could cover things like exclusion of measurements that did not meet predetermined quality criteria, or expressing measurements in a manner that makes them easier to compare. A project looking at obesity may include measurements of body weight, but for this to meaningful you would express this as % predicted, or calculate the body mass index (BMI). This should be stated in the Methods. Finally, you might need to provide the details of the statistical analysis, including the names of any statistical tests and any specialist computer programs you used.

The **Results** section may be relatively short but it is where you put forward your findings. If your research is qualitative, you may need to describe your findings at some length in the text – this is one reason why qualitative reports often have a higher word limit than quantitative reports. As before, subheadings can be helpful and if you have used them to describe different aspects of your project in the methods then you would probably want to report the results in the same manner. In laboratory or clinical science, in particular, you are likely to include tables, charts and illustrations because these are generally a much better means of conveying numerical data than text.

It is important to spend time on considering how best to present your results. Tables are an excellent way of providing a lot of numerical data in a small space. Sometimes you will be able to present all your raw data in tabular form, positioned within the text of your Results, but on other occasions you may need to provide tables that summarise the findings. In this case you may have detailed results tables assembled together in an appendix, where they serve as an archive or data store. If you are unsure about the best option for your data, bear in mind that tables that are too big for a single page rarely work well. In such situations it might be possible to split a table into two or more smaller tables. The layout of a table can make a big difference to the ease with which the information can be assimilated (Box 5.1). The information shown in the two versions of the table are identical but the appearance and readability are much clearer in the second version. In version 1, the title does not stand out clearly from the table itself and the use of gridlines does not help the eye to read across the rows. A redundant column has been accidentally included. In version 2, the title stands out clearly and the use of gaps between different diseases makes the table easier to read, almost inviting the reader to compare the differences between men and women for each disease. When preparing your tables, you may wish to draw particular attention to certain rows, columns or cells. This can be done with judicious use of colour or shading, or by using a larger and/or bold font for the relevant numbers. For example, if you have a table comparing two sets of measurements and their changes after an intervention, you may decide to make all the differences that are statistically significant show up by using a bold font. When presenting numerical data remember to check that the number of significant figures or decimal places is sensible for what is being presented: if you have weighed subjects on scales that record weight to the nearest 0.1 kg it is silly to show mean body weight to three decimal places.

Box 5.1 Comparison of table formatting

Table formatting: version 1						
Longstanding illness by sex, age and condition, 2007, Great Britain						
		All ages	**16–44**	**45–64**	**65–74**	**75+**
		%	**%**	**%**	**%**	**%**
Heart and circulatory system	Men	10.9	1.0	14.7	32.0	33.8
	Women	9.7	1.8	11.0	23.9	27.7
	Both	**10.3**	**1.4**	**12.8**	**27.7**	**30.1**
Heart attack	Men	1.8	0.0	2.2	6.5	5.7
	Women	1.1	0.1	0.8	2.6	5.1
Other heart complaints	Men	3.6	0.3	4.6	10.2	12.1
	Women	2.8	0.6	2.8	6.5	9.6
Hypertension	Men	3.7	0.5	6.0	10.1	7.8
	Women	4.5	0.6	6.0	12.4	9.7
Stroke	Men	0.8	0.0	0.8	2.8	3.8
	Women	0.5	0.1	0.5	1.2	1.9
Other blood vessel/ embolic disorders	Men	0.9	0.2	0.9	2.3	3.9
	Women	0.7	0.4	0.8	1.0	1.1

Table formatting: version 2

Longstanding illness by sex, age and condition, 2007, Great Britain

		All ages	16–44	45–64	65–74	75+
		%	%	%	%	%
Heart and circulatory system	Men	10.9	1.0	14.7	32.0	33.8
	Women	9.7	1.8	11.0	23.9	27.7
	Both	**10.3**	**1.4**	**12.8**	**27.7**	**30.1**
Heart attack	Men	1.8	0.0	2.2	6.5	5.7
	Women	1.1	0.1	0.8	2.6	5.1
Other heart complaints	Men	3.6	0.3	4.6	10.2	12.1
	Women	2.8	0.6	2.8	6.5	9.6
Hypertension	Men	3.7	0.5	6.0	10.1	7.8
	Women	4.5	0.6	6.0	12.4	9.7
Stroke	Men	0.8	0.0	0.8	2.8	3.8
	Women	0.5	0.1	0.5	1.2	1.9
Other blood vessel/ embolic disorders	Men	0.9	0.2	0.9	2.3	3.9
	Women	0.7	0.4	0.8	1.0	1.1

Source: Office for National Statistics (2009) Results from the 2007 General Household Survey, Office for National Statistics. Data available from Table 7.14, located at http://www.ons.gov.uk/ons/publications/re-reference-tables.html?edition=tcm%3A77-53869 (last accessed 22 January 2013).

Tables are an excellent means of providing numerical data in an economical format, but sometimes you will need to present your results in a graph or chart. These visual representations can provide an instant, easy means of conveying information clearly. Figure 5.3 is a simple histogram showing percentages of students achieving different degree classifications, divided into females and males. At a glance the reader can appreciate that the vast majority of students in this cohort were awarded either first class or upper second-class degrees and that the proportions of males and females receiving either class of degree were approximately reversed.

Figure 5.4 shows a scatter plot of individual data points, in this case a measure of lung function plotted against height. It is readily apparent that

Percentage

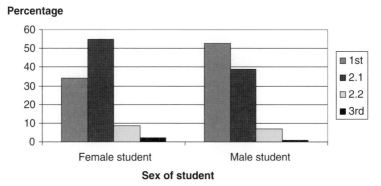

Figure 5.3 Percentage of students with each class of degree, by sex.

lung function increases as the children grow taller, in a manner that looks approximately linear, and that the two groups of children (in this example a group of patients and controls) are different. The extent of the overlap between the two groups and the overall scatter of data can only be appreciated by this type of visual representation.

When working with charts and graphs remember to choose a format that conveys the information as clearly as possible, which usually means avoiding the fancy chart options available in most computer packages. Do not use a pie chart if a histogram is equally effective. Do not display anything in 3D unless it is essential. Make sure each axis is correctly labelled and that the font size of the labelling and the axes can be easily read. If a chart or graph is prepared in a statistical package and imported directly into your dissertation,

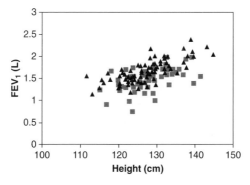

Figure 5.4 FEV_1 against height for primary school children. The patients are shown with square symbols and the controls are triangles.

the labelling or the size of symbols may be inappropriately small when seen on the printed page, so make the adjustments as you prepare the figure. Finally, each figure should have a legend and, where necessary, a footnote to give additional details or to explain an abbreviation.

Your tables and illustrations may be embedded in the text or, for reasons of their size, they may be on a page adjacent to the relevant piece of text. Wherever they occur, it is important to refer to them in the text at the relevant place so that the reader can look at them at the most suitable point in their reading.

The 'Discussion and Conclusions', like the Background and Introduction, may be written in two separate parts or as one section. A **Discussion** section is where you will interpret your findings and place them in the context of other work in the area. The opening paragraph of a Discussion is frequently used to recapitulate the main findings, but this may be superfluous if the project is simple and the Results section is short. You will use the Discussion to state whether the findings supported any hypothesis you may have been working with or not. If not, then you will be expected to explain or speculate why this may have been the case. In interpreting your results you will need to strike a balance between emphasising their importance and the contribution you have made and over-interpreting their significance. It may be helpful to include a subsection on the limitations of the methods. These limitations could be due to many factors, for example

- Equipment not able to detect level of a compound in blood sample below a certain amount
- Measurements made only on healthy young adults – may not be generalisable to older people or patients
- Insufficient number of subjects in the study groups
- If the project was looking at changes over time you may not have had sufficient time to see full effects
- Situations out of your control, for example, accidental defrosting of your samples when freezer broke down
- Repeatability of measurements less good than you predicted, so statistical analysis not clear-cut

When writing about the limitations of your study, try not to give the impression that you are making excuses. Describe the limitation and emphasise what you did to overcome it – or what you would do differently if you had the opportunity.

Elsewhere in your Discussion, you may be comparing your own work with that already published and referring to your own introduction. In your **Conclusions**, you should summarise what contribution your project has made and what has been learned as a result of it. There might be some recommendations arising from your project. You can make suggestions for the next stage of the work or for alternative approaches to investigating the topic. Finishing with a sentence that looks back to the original aim of the project, with a positive feel to it, is a great way to round off your dissertation.

The **References** will almost always be listed at the end of the dissertation. If you have used an electronic reference managing system (as recommended in Chapter 2) it will be easy to populate the text with the reference numbers and produce the list at the end. When you do this, there will be some slight shifting of the text on the page, so complete this task before you give the dissertation its final cosmetic review (see final paragraph of this chapter).

If you are using **Appendices** then these will follow on from the references. Examples of material you may want to include as an appendix include copies of important original documentation, such as ethical approval for your study or written information provided to your study subjects. Another common use of an appendix is as a repository for original data, where this is too much for inclusion in the Results section in its entirety. If you are making an appendix of such material, remember that if it refers to human subjects it should be anonymised, and you (or your supervisor) must keep any associated information that could identify the individual in a secure location.

Maintaining the momentum

Different people take diverse approaches to writing. The most organised will prepare a good plan well ahead of the time that they anticipate beginning to write and will assemble everything they need before sitting down to write. They may write in short bursts or in longer time periods but they will have a schedule to work to. Others will be more spontaneous in their writing and will sit down at their keyboard and get started when other tasks can be put to one side, hoping or expecting that their writing will flow. Plenty of others will procrastinate until a deadline is too close to ignore and then stay up half the night in desperation. Students in this last group are the most likely to let themselves down in the production of their dissertation, not to mention suffering from lack of sleep! Whichever category you fall in to, unless you are in the throes of a creative episode, you will experience periods when the writing seems to just dry up. This is commonly known as 'writer's block' and can delay progress and cause undue stress. There are different strategies you can employ so that you do not lose momentum.

Remember that your dissertation does not require only the text. If writing is not going well, do something else that is essential for your dissertation. Such tasks might include the following:

1 Assemble any illustrations and photographs you plan to include. If any of them require the publisher's permission to reproduce, send off those e-mails.

2 Work on any diagrams and figures you are preparing yourself and ensure you know where they will be positioned in the text.

3 Prepare the titles and write the footnotes to your figures and illustrations. Make sure that these explain clearly what is shown so that they can 'stand alone' as far as possible.

4 If you are planning to include any appendices then prepare them.

Completing some of these tasks might be sufficient to stimulate you to recommence writing your text.

If you have done what you can to make progress on 'non-text-writing' tasks and you **need** to continue writing, what you do might depend on why you have got writer's block. If you have been focusing on something complex that requires a great deal of detail, and you feel that you 'can't see the wood for the trees', leave that section for another day and begin to write a part of a completely different chapter. For example, although you may not have completed your analysis (and therefore you do not have your final results), you may be fairly confident of your main message and be able to write part of your Discussion section sooner than you might have thought possible. When you return to the section that proved so difficult after a break of a day or two, you may well find that what you need to write has suddenly become clear.

Sometimes you find that you cannot express what it is you want to say in a fluent style. The words just desert you. When this happens, try writing down what you want to say as if you were speaking to a fellow student who had asked you to talk about your project. Do not be concerned at this stage with structuring your sentences or paragraphs or writing 'scientifically' – just focus on getting the important points down on the screen. Nobody except you will read this draft, so it does not matter if it is badly written. When you have finished what you need to say, then you can go back, reorder the points into a logical sequence and then revise the standard of writing so that it is properly structured, grammatically correct and reads well. Your writer's block just went away.

One tip to reduce the chance of writer's block striking again is not to leave a writing session when you have completed a chapter or section. It is then much more difficult to get back into the swing of writing again. Instead, write down the first couple of sentences of another section so that when you return to your keyboard you are not facing a blank screen.

There may be times when you think that the task is overwhelming and that you will never be able to write a dissertation. This is when a bit of maths can help. Imagine the word count for your dissertation is 10 000 words, and you have just 6 weeks to write it. If you want to keep your weekends free, that leaves you 30 days of writing. If you wrote the same amount each day, you would need to write just 333 words each day to complete the dissertation. That is roughly the equivalent of the last three paragraphs, which is hardly a monumental daily task. Of course nobody would suggest that writing 300–350 words per day is a good approach to completing a dissertation, and it ignores all the associated tasks and the revisions you will need to complete, but it suddenly makes the dissertation appear achievable.

Attention to detail: presentation, grammar and spelling

In some institutions a proportion of the marks will be allocated for general presentation, standard of written English, grammar and spelling. You may think that this is unfair, since you want to be judged on your scientific achievements, but a slovenly presentation can only detract from good science. If you annoy the reader by writing sentences with no verbs, or by misuse of punctuation, lack of numbering system to figures, or similar crimes against the language you will not only lose those marks allocated for presentation but may lead the examiner into thinking everything else is sloppy.

A fluent scientific writing style does not come naturally to everyone but it can be developed and cultivated. Many years ago all scientific reports were written using only the passive voice; this is no longer considered de rigueur. Using the active voice can, however, make reading a report rather tiresome, particularly in the 'Methods' section. Consider the following short passage:

> We first calibrated the whatsit before we connected it to the thingummy. Next, we added the blue liquid and waited 30 minutes before we took a few drops and placed them on a microscope slide. We examined the slide at × 40 magnification for evidence of cellular uptake.

The word 'we' appears five times. A more streamlined passage would be:

> We calibrated the whatsit prior to connecting it to the thingummy and adding the blue liquid. After waiting for 30 minutes a few drops were placed on a microscope slide and examined at × 40 magnification for evidence of cellular uptake.

In the second passage the same information is conveyed in two sentences rather than three. Sentence length is important. A passage in which **all** the sentences are very brief is usually very clear but can resemble a primary school reading book. In contrast, overly long sentences are difficult to assimilate and the reader may lose the thread of meaning. Avoid using sentences of more than 40–50 words, and aim for prose incorporating sentences of contrasting length. Remember that information in a series of short sentences (such as a description of a series of actions) may be better conveyed using bullet points or in a flow diagram. Take the opportunity to read parts of dissertations written by students in a previous cohort and form a judgement about what makes some passages easier to read and assimilate than others.

Most people will use a word-processing package that incorporates a spellchecker and a grammar checker. These are invaluable. The wiggly red lines that appear under a word can draw your attention to the occasional typing error or to an incorrect spelling. Despite their usefulness, spellcheckers are not infallible, particularly when two different words have very similar spellings. For example

The college principal commended all the students for their hard work.

The student calculated the optimum concentration from first principles.

Both these sentences are correct but if the spellings of principal/principle had been interchanged they would have been meaningless. The spellchecker would not have alerted the writer to the mistake. Some words are spelled differently according to whether they are being used as a noun, verb or adjective. Consider the examples below:

Mucus is a sticky substance secreted by **mucous** glands.

Before the newborn animal begins to **breathe** air, its lungs are full of liquid. The first **breath** will introduce air into the lung and a stable lung volume will develop shortly afterwards.

The student completely forgot about football **practice** because he was too busy **practising** his spoken presentation.

Again, the spellchecker will not help you here. To guard against such errors you should ask someone to read a portion of your work specifically to look for inappropriate spelling or grammatical constructions. Ask someone that you know writes well themselves, who is also familiar with your topic, so they are likely to detect such errors at the outset.

If you are a student for whom English is not your first language, you may think you have more difficulty than others over written English. This is not necessarily true, because you may well have studied English grammar, whereas students educated in the UK probably did not! Asking someone to read your work may be particularly valuable, however, and you should find out if your institution offers support for students in your situation. What you cannot expect is that someone will rewrite your dissertation for you; it should be your own work.

Avoiding plagiarism

Plagiarism means taking somebody else's work and passing it off as if it were your own. At its worst it involves copying, or cutting and pasting, someone else's work into your own document without any acknowledgement. This is cheating. All universities regard this as a very serious offence and their codes of conduct will reflect this.

To reflect this, it is common practice for students to be asked for an electronic version of their dissertation at the time when they hand in a hard copy. This has to be accompanied by a declaration that the two versions are identical (although the electronic copy may sometimes be submitted without the references, and any illustrations that require huge files may also sometimes need to be cut out). The university will submit the electronic versions to plagiarism detection software that will give an index of similarity; that is, it will provide an estimate of what proportion of the work closely resembles published work or other student's submissions. By itself, this index is not especially useful. The Methods section of one project may have a lot of overlap with other work, because the techniques used may be identical and the ways of describing them are limited. One or more people will be given the task of viewing the reports and comparing sections of your dissertation with other published or archived materials and form a judgement; if they have any concerns they will almost certainly seek input from other colleagues. Because accusations of plagiarism are viewed so seriously they would only be made if there was strong evidence, confirmed by more than one individual.

Few students will deliberately set out to plagiarise someone else's work, but many will be anxious that if they depend heavily on prior publications in formulating their own dissertations, their work could be considered as plagiarism. It is likely that your institution will have guidelines or run tutorials on how to avoid plagiarism and these should clarify for you exactly what does or does not constitute plagiarism. The following guidelines should help:

- When taking notes, make sure you record the source of the information so you can reference it appropriately, and include it in your reference managing system (see Chapter 2).
- If you want or need to use the exact words from published work, then use quotation marks. A precise definition, for example, could not usually be given without quoting it 'word for word'. The reference should be provided

in the format used throughout your dissertation but is shown in full for the following example.

> 'SIDS is defined as the sudden unexpected death of an infant < 1 year of age, with onset of the fatal episode apparently occurring during sleep, that remains unexplained after a thorough investigation, including performance of a complete autopsy and review of the circumstances of death and the clinical history'. Krous HF et al., Sudden Infant Death Syndrome and Unclassified Sudden Infant Deaths: A Definitional and Diagnostic Approach. *Pediatrics* 2004;114:234–238.

• When paraphrasing another article, ensure that your writing makes clear what ideas, evidence or data come from another source. Consider the two related paragraphs below, about ethnic differences in lung function.

> 'Comparing our results to studies conducted in India, white children had lung volumes approximately 17% larger than Indian children.[28][29] The Asian children living in Leicester had lung volumes approximately 6% greater than those in India. The reasons for this probably relate to socio-economic factors including nutrition and exposure to pollution, although genetic differences within subsets of the same ethnic or racial groups cannot be ruled out. Socioeconomic status influences pulmonary function in adults,[30] but ethnic differences remain even when the study groups are restricted to young adults of similar socio-economic status, [4] or when adjustments are made for socioeconomic status and level of education. [19]'
>
> *Original paragraph taken from Whittaker et al. 2005 'Do chest wall dimensions explain ethnicity-related differences in lung function in children?' Arch Dis Child 90: F423–F428.*
>
> 'Lung volumes in Asian children are smaller than those of white children. This is likely to be so because of socioeconomic differences such as nutrition and the extent of pollution in the local environment. Studies in adults have shown effects of socioeconomic status on pulmonary function (ref) although these do not completely account for ethnic differences (ref). Genetic differences cannot, however, be ruled out.'
>
> This paragraph is plagiarised. The ideas expressed in the original work have been reformulated without reference to the source document. The person responsible for the plagiarised paragraph has quoted the same two references mentioned in the original, but has not given any credit to the author (Whittaker) for her ideas or interpretation. Altering the order of the words or introducing minor changes in phrasing does not negate the plagiarism.

• Some information that you include in your dissertation may be so well known or accepted that there is no need to reference the source – indeed, sources may have become lost in the mists of time or be so plentiful that you cannot realistically cite them. Omitting to cite references when they would clearly be important is at best poor scholarship and may spill over into plagiarism. Consider the following paragraph and decide at which point you would expect to position a reference:

> 'The association between cigarette smoking and lung cancer is well-known, and the impact of passive smoking on the respiratory health of non-smokers is becoming increasingly accepted. The impact of maternal smoking during pregnancy on the respiratory system of the unborn child, though less well-known, is significant. Ante-natal exposure to cigarette smoke has been shown to be associated with changes in lung mechanics in the infant, increased risk of respiratory infection in the first six months of life, and increased risk of cot death.'

The first sentence does not necessarily need any referencing because the information is widespread within the public domain. A reference to a good review article would be appropriate at the end of the second sentence. The three associations listed in the third sentence are highly specific and references to the original studies should be included.

Allowing sufficient time for each aspect of your dissertation (planning, reading, note taking, drafting and revising) will allow you to think clearly about what you are committing to paper, so that the final work is undoubtedly your own, meaning that you avoid plagiarism. It also allows you time for revising your written work so that the final product is as good as you can make it.

Revisions, revisions

Allowing time for revision of your dissertation is essential if you want it to be outstanding. There may be more than one revision of certain parts, depending on the complexity of the writing, the time available, and (perhaps) your supervisor's attitude.

The purpose of a revision is to improve on what has been written already. Consequently, when you have just completed a chapter or a section you will not be in the best frame of mind to recognise its flaws or see where it could be made clearer. Put the section to one side, ideally for a few days, so that when you read it again it is fresh to you and you can spot the gaps, illogical ordering of paragraphs, sentences that make no sense at all, charts that do not display what you really intended, and other things that need your attention.

Input from your supervisor can be invaluable here. Before asking for this, make sure you understand what level of support you can expect. If your supervisor is also one of your examiners, then he or she may have restrictions on what support they can give (e.g. it may be acceptable for them to comment on the plan, and/or on a first draft, but no more than that). Find out what your supervisor expects from you, and what their preferred way of working is. For example, ask if he or she prefers smaller sections at a time or wants to see bigger sections. Find out at the outset what sort of 'turnaround' time you can expect. This is important because if they expect to have your work for a week or more, then that could severely restrict the time remaining for you to implement any suggestions they might make. Ask your supervisor if they would prefer the hard copy or the electronic copy, and how they prefer to give suggestions. Some people will prefer electronic versions and they will add annotations and return your document, whereas others prefer to write by hand on a hard copy. An appointment where you meet with your supervisor to discuss their recommendations is excellent because it enables him or her to expand on something they have written and you can ask supplementary questions. If possible, make commitments with your supervisor whereby you deliver a given piece of work on a set date and agree upon a follow-up meeting for receiving your feedback.

Sometimes you will need to make major revisions, such as at times when you may have exceeded your allowed word count by a huge amount, or when you decide you need a major restructuring of the dissertation. On other occasions, changes will be much smaller and may just require including an extra diagram or rephrasing a few sentences. Word processing packages make the task relatively straightforward but you will still need time to work out exactly how to rewrite a troublesome paragraph. Finding exactly the right words to express what you need to say is the skill of writing well.

As you work your way through the various iterations and revisions of your dissertation, make sure that each version is saved with a filename that includes the date so that you can keep track of changes. Always make sure you have at least one secure backup, because computers fail, memory sticks get lost and laptops get stolen. Your institution will certainly have automated backups of the central computer system so, even if you prefer to work on a private laptop, make it a habit to e-mail the dissertation to your institutional account each time you have worked on it.

When you have completed the dissertation in full you will be in the position of making a final revision. If possible, ask another person to read it in its entirety and give you feedback. Go through it again yourself and check that you have implemented all the earlier changes you required. Reread your concluding paragraphs, in particular, as these will 'stay with' the reader when they close the dissertation. Do they make a positive statement or convey a sense of deflation? Without over-interpreting your findings or overemphasising their importance, try to finish on a positive note.

Lastly, check every detail of any instructions you have relating to the dissertation. You may be asked to put the final word count on the title page and this could easily be overlooked when you are overcome with relief at having finished. Pay particular attention to the abstract. Check that the reference formatting is correct, both within the text and where they are listed at the end. Check that the contents pages are accurate and the pages are numbered. When you think it is perfect, take time to go through it on screen, page by page. You are checking it for overall cosmetic effect. Make sure that a table has not been shifted so that it cuts across two pages, or that a diagram has become detached from its legend. Avoid having a heading at the bottom of a page if the subsequent text begins on the next page. Save the final version, and print it off. Even at this late stage, do not relax your guard, just in case the printer runs out of ink part-way through, or treats you to a paper jam. Finally, your dissertation will be ready to be bound and submitted and you can relax.

SUMMARY

Start planning your dissertation as early as possible ensuring that it meets with the requirements of your institution relating to length, presentation and so on. Drafting the 'Contents' pages at the outset will help you to structure the dissertation. While generally working within the accepted pattern of Introduction, Aims, Methods, Results, Discussion and Conclusions, ensure that the structure is one that is most logical for the reader. Make good use of subheadings. Figures, charts, tables and illustrations add greatly to the quality of a dissertation.

Avoid plagiarism at all costs.

Be aware that many people go through periods of 'writer's block' when they find it difficult to make progress. There are strategies for overcoming this, including focusing on other aspects of preparing a dissertation.

Pay attention to detail and leave time for final revisions so that the final result is something you can be proud of.

Chapter 6 **Maximising impact**

CHAPTER OVERVIEW

While student research projects are written up as dissertations, submitted and marked, the enthusiastic and motivated student will seek out other ways to get the most out of the experience of his or her project. This may include spoken or poster presentations within the institution or beyond. The chapter explains what makes for a powerful presentation, and how to prepare for them. Suggestions are made about where a student might seek out their own presentation opportunities, and where a poster might later be placed for maximum impact. Other self-made opportunities for publicising the work such as a blog or a press release are suggested, although it must be emphasised that any dissemination of research findings must only be made with the full consent and approval of the supervisor.

Maximising impact in the context of a research project can mean different things. It might refer to the impact that the process has on you, the student, for your learning and whatever you may gain personally from the experience. It could refer to what you can do to promote your own research to the widest audience, or it could be about making yourself as an individual stand out from the crowd. Clearly there is a lot of overlap in these three areas, particularly the last two, since if your research is high profile, so will you be!

Think back to Chapter 1 and the reasons why you are doing your project. Remind yourself exactly what you want to get out of the process. In many cases, it will contribute to the mark or grade you get at the end of the academic year, and in some cases it will determine the classification of your degree. Some individuals may feel that this is all they can commit to, because

---

How to do your Research Project: A Guide for Students in Medicine and the Health Sciences, First Edition. Caroline Beardsmore.
© 2013 John Wiley & Sons, Ltd. Published 2013 by John Wiley & Sons, Ltd.

their personal circumstances preclude much else. The majority of students, however, can take things to a higher level and add lasting value to the research project.

Promoting your research

The two best recognised means of promoting your research are (i) talking about it and (ii) writing about it! A poster presentation is a hybrid of these. A spoken presentation also involves skills other than speaking because you will usually be expected to produce slides to illustrate your talk. Your institution may require you to present your work verbally or in a poster format as a part of your coursework and, of course, you will be writing up your work as a part of the assessment. We will consider the approaches to spoken presentations and posters in turn.

Giving a good spoken presentation

Many students are filled with fear and trepidation at the prospect of giving a spoken presentation. Even people who are experienced at spoken presentations and would be considered confident speakers are likely to have a degree of apprehension under certain circumstances, and this should be regarded as normal. The key to a great presentation, whatever the degree of experience, is proper preparation. This takes time, so start early and allow time for rehearsal and subsequent changes.

Know your audience

This may seem obvious but not everyone thinks this through. At the end of your talk you want every member of the audience to take away your main message and be able to identify what they have learned. If you are talking to your student peers you should give them enough background so that they will understand your research topic and why it is important. Although your audience is likely to include academic staff who are experts in your area, they will be noting if your talk is comprehensible to your peers. If you are presenting at a specialist conference, the level of background information you provide will clearly be different and you will probably be able to talk in greater depth. Surprisingly, talking to a lay audience can be the most challenging. Be especially careful about the use of abbreviations or specialist language; you should speak about 'myocardial infarction' when talking to an audience who understands the term, but this could alienate a lay audience who would better understand the term 'heart attack'. If you are not sure which term to use, you could explain the professional term at the outset and then continue to use it thereafter. If you are talking about any medical conditions beware of saying anything that could be construed in a way that makes you look uncaring or callous: there may be someone in the audience who is personally affected in some way by the condition under discussion.

Plan the time and construct the talk

Often you will know how long you are expected to speak for and you must tailor your presentation accordingly. Do not fall into the trap of trying to cram too much information into the time available or you risk either going so fast through your presentation that nobody can follow it, which is a waste of their time and yours, or else you find yourself still talking beyond the end of the allotted time. In this case the chairperson will be obliged to curtail your talk or the session will overrun, neither of which will reflect well on you. If there are several parts to your project and you do not have the time to cover all of them then accept the reality of the situation. You could begin your talk in this manner:

> I'm going to present my work investigating the use of complementary medicines in the treatment of allergy. I will be discussing the different types of medicines available for several allergic conditions. A separate part of my project focused on **attitudes** to allergies but I do not have time to cover this topic now. If anyone has a particular interest in this I'll be pleased to tell you about it during the coffee break.

On another occasion you may have the opportunity to talk about your project in a setting where there is no requirement to keep to a precise time. This might be at a research group seminar or regular meeting where timings are more relaxed. Whether your time allocation is strict or not, you should consider the overall balance of your talk. This means thinking about the emphasis you place on different sections, typically Background, Aims, Methods, Results and Discussion. Talking to your supervisor will help you get the balance right. If your work is at an early stage and you have few results, it may be appropriate to concentrate on the details of your methods. If you are presenting your completed project at a specialist conference and your methods are standardised and in widespread use, do not spend precious time describing them.

In constructing your talk you might find it helpful to think of it as sending a friend on a journey. You know the starting point, and where you want to end up, but you need to plan the best route so that your friend can move from one landmark to another without getting lost on the journey. You have to plan the talk so that you present the information in a logical manner, making use of spoken and visual signposts to move from one section to another. Make sure that you round off the talk in such a way that the audience knows when you have brought things to a conclusion. Exactly how you construct your talk will be a matter of personal preference coupled with the nature of the topic. If your talk is in the nature of a review, where you have not performed any experimental work of your own, it may not be appropriate to work through the Methods, Results, Discussion triad that is often at the heart of presentations. You may start with a blank sheet of paper, write the title of your talk on the middle, and then jot down all the things you want to include linked into a web or a mind map before you work out the best means of ordering what you want to say. Alternatively, you may want to work out your opening lines first, and then plan the talk in a linear manner, step-by-step and slide-by-slide. Some people will move straight to designing their slides using a package such as PowerPoint and make use of the facility to add notes as an **aide-memoire** to the speaker. The disadvantage of this approach is that the presentation can tend to drive the message, which is getting things the wrong way round. Knowing what you want to convey before moving to slide design is generally considered a more successful approach. Having said that, there is no universal correct manner of preparation – it depends on what works for you. What is **not** a good plan is to write out exactly what you want to say, word-for-word, because reading or memorising a script will tend to make you speak in a monotone. If you 'lose your thread' or have an unexpected interruption you may find it more difficult to pick up where you left off. You may want to write out an occasional sentence if there is something that is complicated to explain so that you can refer to it if you need to. Knowing that you have the key sentence written out may give you an added confidence when you give your talk.

When you have worked out the main points of your talk and the order you want to introduce them in, you are likely to move to planning your slides.

Prepare your slides

It is rare to hear a talk on any topic, especially a scientific topic, which is not accompanied by a slide presentation. Until the advent of applications such as PowerPoint, slides had to be prepared and mounted by hand, which was a lengthy process and therefore usually only done for formal presentations where a slide projector was available. The overhead projector was something of a poor relation, but did allow images hand-drawn or printed onto sheets of acetate, to be projected. In recent years the availability of programs and the low cost of projectors mean that slides are used at every opportunity. In preparing your slides you must consider what you will say when each slide is projected, and how many slides you expect to use, given the time available for you to speak. The number of slides that is 'reasonable' cannot be readily judged because the time required for the audience to assimilate the information on a slide depends entirely on their complexity. Excluding the

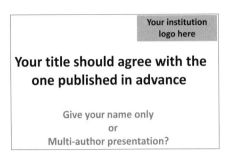

Figure 6.1 Example of a title slide for a spoken presentation.

title and acknowledgement slides, if the number of your slides is more than 1.5 × the number of minutes you have to speak you should consider seriously if you are trying to pack too much information into the presentation. When you are building your presentation, you may find that you have far more slides than you will be able to use and then you will have to be selective and dispense with some of them. As you build your presentation, you are likely to concentrate primarily on getting the content onto the slide and to give less thought to the impression on your audience. You should try to see things through the eyes – and ears – of others and pay attention to what each slide conveys. Consider the following examples as you plan your own presentation.

Your title slide (Figure 6.1) will remind the audience what they are about to hear and tell them who they are listening to. Outside your own department you will probably want to have your institutional logo displayed, and you may choose to include it in all your slides. If you are presenting a piece of research on behalf of several people then all their names will be included. By convention the person giving the talk will be named first on the slide.

If you are following a format of Background or Introduction, Aims, Methods, Results and so on, then it may be helpful to provide these headings to the audience (Figure 6.2). You may have several slides in each section, and

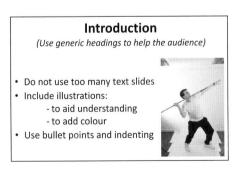

Figure 6.2 Example of a slide layout suitable for introducing a topic.

numbering them (Methods (1), Methods (2), etc.) helps you to keep them in order as you are planning your talk. Using text on a slide is a great way of helping the speaker to cover all the main points, in a sensible order, but if it turns into a presentation where the speaker reads the slides to the audience it can be a rather stultifying experience. Use illustrations to enliven what you are saying.

Figure 6.3 is a slide used to display a particular way of analysing recordings, so it appears in a 'Methods' section. Since it is an illustration taken directly from a computer screen it adds a certain immediacy to the presentation, but each part of the figure will need explaining to the audience. Sometimes you will want the listener to look only at one part of the figure, so you may need to introduce this slide by saying something like 'Please ignore the three small graphs on the right, and concentrate first on the single recording in the top left of the slide. . . ' A complex slide like this may take between 1 and 2 minutes for the audience to fully appreciate what you are showing them: make sure you give them sufficient time before moving on to the next.

With complex slides of this nature, use the laser pointer to advantage by directing the audience to what you want them to look at. If your hand is unsteady when using the pointer, try resting your elbow on the lectern or, if there is no suitable furniture handy, use your spare hand to hold the wrist steady when using the pointer.

Figure 6.4 is typical of a slide from the Results part of a research presentation. In this example the symbols that represent different patient groups are differentiated by shape and colour, but are probably a bit too large for the viewer to see how one group compares with another. Think about how the slide will look when projected onto the screen. If possible, expand the proportion of the slide occupied by the data points. Currently the area of the graph is approximately one quarter of the whole area: repositioning the box that contains the key to symbols would allow this to be increased.

Again, a Results section may involve use of tables (Figure 6.5). The table in Figure 6.5 has six columns and seven rows, probably rather too much for most presentations. The use of a highlight to focus attention on the bottom row may help at the time of the talk.

The menu of different slide styles available can suggest the means of presenting your work. The two-panel format can be used to list advantages and disadvantages (Figure 6.6) or to compare two groups, for example, patients in a randomised controlled trial. Alternatively one panel can be used to provide an illustration, as in Figure 6.2. Make use of video clips if it adds to what you are saying but make sure the clip will 'run' on the computer you will be using beforehand. It is a bit of a let-down if you have to stand in front of the audience and tell them what they would see if only the equipment functioned as you wanted it to!

Give the audience time to fully understand
each slide. In this example they would
need to be told the axes on each graph.

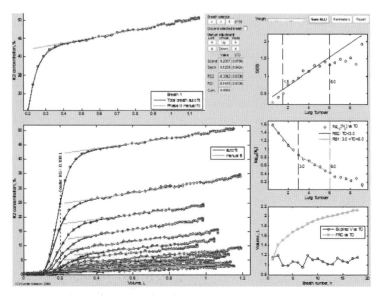

Figure 6.3 Example of a complex slide that will require the speaker to take plenty of
time to explain to the audience.

Here, labelling and font size are reasonable
but symbols are a bit big to be distinguishable

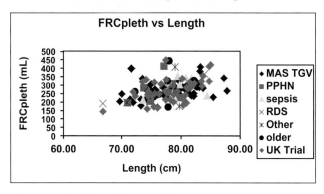

Figure 6.4 Example of a 'Results' section slide.

Results
(Try to incorporate tables and charts)

Measurement	Predicted Value	Lower limit	Upper limit	Baseline	SR
FRCp (L)	1.72	1.24	2.2	2.75	3.56
TLC (L)	3.31	2.66	3.97	3.85	1.36
RV (L)	0.9	0.48	1.31	2.43	6.11
VC (L)	2.49	1.92	3.05	1.42	−3.09
RV%TLC	24.7	16.9	32.5	63	8.06
Rtot (kPa*s/L)	0.24	0.11	0.37	1.48	15.41

- Do not put too many rows or columns in your tables.
- Use colours or highlights to emphasize what you want the audience to notice.

Figure 6.5 Example of a table of results.

Figure 6.6 has used bullet points, which provide an easy way of listing points you want to cover. Try not to be over-reliant on bullet points. This slide is functional, but its appearance is distinctly boring.

While the technology can certainly help you to produce a great presentation, do not fall into the trap of using every gizmo on the toolbar or choosing some whacky colour or design combinations (Figure 6.7). Often the simplest styles work best. Be consistent in how you make the transition from one slide to the next so that your audience is not distracted, waiting to see if the next transition is coming from the top left of the screen or if it will be a gradual fade-out. When you reach your penultimate slide, refer back to the Aims of

Take advantage of the technology

Advantages of this application:
- Choice of layouts
- Easy and intuitive to build a presentation
- Can add video clips, sound, animations
- Can be revised and updated at the last moment

Disadvantages:
- Temptation to use all the tricks
- Style over substance
- Over-reliance on putting text on slides
- Can be revised and updated at the last moment, which can add to stress!

Figure 6.6 Two-panel slide design can be useful to compare advantages and disadvantages.

Conclusions

*(Again, a generic heading helps the
audience to know when you are finishing)*

- The colour combination and style of this slide is a distraction
- Be careful about using background styles and colours, especially if your content is colourful
- What works well with a text slide can spoil your charts
- Think about font styles and size that best help the audience read your slides

Figure 6.7 Avoid backgrounds that could distract from the content of your slides or make them difficult to read.

your work, probably introduced early on in your presentation, and explain how these have been fulfilled or not.

A final slide acknowledging the help and support of colleagues or outside bodies, particularly those that have funded the work, will be appropriate at meetings outside your own institution but may be rather superfluous in a local setting (Figure 6.8). If there are more than one or two named individuals, do not read them all aloud but allow the audience to absorb the names as you thank them for their attention.

As you prepare your slides you will be referring to the notes you made at the start of the planning process, and you will be working out what you want

Example of
Acknowledgements

- My supervisor Dr Brown
- Senior Technician Jack Williams
- All colleagues in the Physiology Laboratories
- The Billbloggs Charity for financial support

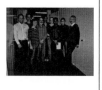

Figure 6.8 A final slide of acknowledgements is a good way of rounding off a formal presentation.

to say. You may make notes to yourself using the facility within PowerPoint, so that they are linked to the slide being displayed as you speak. Alternatively you may prefer to make notes by hand, using one record card per slide. This may seem rather old-fashioned but it works well. Keep your cards together by punching a hole in each card and inserting a treasury tag, because then you can rearrange them if you alter the order of your slides and if you drop the whole lot they will not get out of order! Something that I use myself is to print out the slides (usually six to a page) when the talk is prepared and hand-write my brief notes below each image. This has the advantage that you can readily see which slides are coming up next, and can make a smooth verbal transition from one slide to another. This is much more professional than changing slides and having to try and disguise the fact that you were not sure what was coming up next! These printouts of your slides can be protected in a clear plastic sleeve and linked together with treasury tags for the reasons indicated above.

Rehearse and respond to feedback

If your presentation is to your own small group of colleagues, without a strict time schedule, you may decide that it is not essential to spend a lot of time on rehearsing your talk. Your supervisor will guide you on this. If you are talking in a more formal setting, particularly outside your own department, rehearsals are important to make a really good presentation.

When you have prepared your slides you can start to practise your presentation. You are most likely to start doing this by yourself, in front of your computer. Do not just 'go through it in your head' but speak aloud as you will do on the day. Allow time for anyone seeing each slide for the first time to understand what is being conveyed. The first time you go through your talk, write down the time that you started, and then do not look at any watch or clock until you have finished. By doing that, you will get a better idea of whether you might be able to extend what you say or if you need to shorten the talk. After going through your presentation by yourself, and before spending more time on polishing it, have a rehearsal in front of other people. Your supervisor should be involved, but where possible others should participate. The whole idea is that your colleagues will make suggestions to improve both the content of the talk and your presentation. Be prepared for them to ask for new slides to be included, existing slides to be altered or omitted, and for a change in the order of the slides. Have a notebook handy so that you can write down what is suggested. If the suggestions are very radical you might feel as if all your preparatory work was a waste of time, but you should instead regard it as an invaluable learning experience.

It is likely that you will recognise many of the suggestions made to you as ones that will improve your presentation and you will be pleased to accept them. Sometimes different people who hear your rehearsal will have alternative suggestions for your talk and you will need to discuss the merits of both approaches. On occasion you will disagree with what is suggested. Do not be afraid to express your own opinions, but if you find them at odds with everyone else's then think carefully before ignoring the advice of others.

Whether you have a second rehearsal will depend on the extent of the changes to the presentation, the prestige of the meeting at which you will be speaking and your own level of confidence. Having a second rehearsal will probably boost your confidence and help with the timing required for each slide. At a first rehearsal, some minor points may have gone unmentioned because of the overriding need to change the shape of the talk and suggest alterations to the slides. At a second rehearsal the audience can suggest small improvements to what you say, and any distracting habits (e.g. saying 'um' too often, or continually shuffling your notes) can be addressed. It is worth asking specifically about these, as your colleagues may be reticent about telling you about your personal habits.

One important function of a rehearsal is to identify the possible questions you may get asked, so that you can prepare your answers. Sometimes you may find that a slide you had prepared and then set aside might help to answer a likely question; reserve slides can be kept at the end of your presentation so they can be used during question time if needed.

Once your presentation is complete and you have rehearsed it with colleagues and they have indicated that it is good, you have no further need of rehearsal. You may want to run through it again, just to become more slick and confident on the podium if you are presenting at an important conference.

Delivering your spoken presentation

If the rehearsals have served their purpose you should have no trouble in delivering a good presentation. Nevertheless, there are some tips to help things run smoothly, particularly if you are speaking at an unfamiliar venue and as part of a conference where your talk is grouped with several others.

i. Read any instructions and follow them exactly. You may be asked to e-mail your presentation in advance so the slides can be preloaded or told where to take your slides ahead of the session where you are speaking.

ii. Arrive in plenty of time to get your presentation loaded or to check it if it was sent ahead. It is likely that you will have your presentation on a memory stick. Consider having a backup available in case of a disaster, either on a separate memory stick or e-mailed to yourself in a way that you could download it from anywhere.

iii. Check out the room where you will be speaking before the audience arrive. Familiarise yourself with any controls on the podium, such as the laser pointer and how to dim the lights. If there is a microphone, see if it is fixed or one that clips to your clothing. Take note of where the person chairing the meeting will be sitting.

iv. The chairperson is likely to arrive before the session as he or she will want to make sure that all the speakers are present. If you have never met, introduce yourself to the chairperson and the other speakers.

v. Sit somewhere near the front so you do not waste time with a long walk to the podium. When your turn arrives, go over to the podium. It is customary to begin with a greeting to the chairperson and the audience, then away you go!

As you communicate with the audience they will be taking in the information visually from your slides, and aurally by listening to what you are saying. Do check that the slide being displayed on the screen behind you is the one that you are talking about, and use the pointer when you need to draw attention to particular things, such as specific cells on a histological slide. You should be aware that laser pointers should never be pointed directly at an audience as they can injure the eyes. Use them only to point to specific things on your slide and do not fall into the habit of sending the coloured dot whizzing around the screen in a frenzy. If you have control of the light levels, adjust these so that your slides are seen to best advantage but the audience are not sitting in near-total darkness.

The verbal aspect of the presentation will be successful if you speak fairly slowly, clearly and using the microphone if one is provided. If you turn to look at the screen, this will not matter if the microphone is clipped to your collar but if it is a fixed device your voice will suddenly be lost. As you deliver your talk, do not be afraid to introduce pauses from time to time. These will give the audience time to absorb what you have been saying or to look at what is on the screen. Without trying to give an Oscar-winning performance, use your voice carefully to give added emphasis where needed. If you speak in a boring monotone, even those members of the audience who stay awake may not realise the excitement of what you are saying. This is one very good reason **not** to read your talk. If English is not your first language it may be a particular temptation to read (or learn) your talk but it never gives a good effect. A more spontaneous presentation, even with some errors, will give a better result. Do try to look at the audience as much as possible as this enhances the feeling of a conversation. If you find it hard to look at a particular person, set your eyes somewhere about two-thirds back from the front row and this will give the impression that you are looking at the audience.

After concluding your talk, the chairperson is likely to invite questions. As these cannot be entirely predicted, it can be the most anxious part of the procedure. If the chairperson is good in this role, he or she will make sure that the question was heard properly by everyone and that you have the chance to answer. If you need a moment to prepare your response, take the time. If you are not clear about what is being asked, then check with the questioner before attempting to answer. If you do not know the answer to the question, it is usually acceptable to say so, but you may be in a position to offer a guess or to speculate. If this is the case, make it clear that you are proffering a speculative response. If your supervisor or other senior colleague is in the audience they may be able to supplement any answers you have given, but try and field all the questions yourself. This presentation is your moment of glory; make the most of it!

Preparing a poster presentation

Poster presentations are way of showcasing your project in a way that interested individuals can glean the main message in a relatively short time. The poster should be able to be viewed as a stand-alone item, but in many poster sessions the presenter will be expected to be present over a set period of time so that others can ask questions. Although each person that views the poster may not spend more than a few minutes looking at it, a good poster takes time to prepare.

When preparing a poster, you will have to consider the likely audience, and the content and appearance of the poster itself. A poster designed for a highly specialised scientific meeting will not be the same as one aiming to convey a health education message. We will assume for present purposes that you are preparing a poster for sharing with other students and staff involved with the research project part of your curriculum. How will you set about it?

First you should read any instructions about things such as the final size of the poster and any guidance about printing. Posters are frequently produced using Microsoft PowerPoint. The best effect is achieved if the poster is printed by your institutional print department on a single piece of paper (which can be laminated if the poster is likely to sustain damage or if it needs to last a long time). If you are not going to the expense of printing a large poster professionally, it can be printed off in several pieces of A4 paper that can then be mounted on a board to give the effect of a large poster. The advantage of PowerPoint is that you can resize objects and move then around very easily until you are happy with the appearance.

Before beginning to work on the appearance, plan the content of the poster. There will be a title and the names of those sharing in the research, usually at the top. If this poster relates only to your own work, then it may be appropriate for you to be the single author, but in this case you should indicate somewhere the name of your supervisor. Beyond that, the content will be dictated by the nature of your project. If you are doing a laboratory project it is likely that you will provide some background, a clearly stated aim, a methods section and your results and conclusions. A library project may be a very different composition. Whatever you decide as the pattern for your poster, try and think of a thread running through the various parts, so that they link in a logical manner. Next, decide what will best convey the information in each section, whether this is a text, a diagram, a flow chart, a figure or a combination. Remember, a picture is worth a thousand words and will draw the audience to your poster far more than any text. Now move to thinking about the poster layout and put on the title and the author's names and departmental affiliation. You may want to add an institutional or departmental logo. Prepare and assemble what you will include that is not pure text, positioning them on the poster in roughly the regions where you expect them to end up. Only then prepare the text that you will use, typing it up in various 'boxes' and putting them on the poster.

When you have created a rough draft of your poster layout, you should consider carefully what you can do to make it stand out and attract attention, but also encourage the viewer to read and study each part and leave with increased knowledge and understanding. Consider the examples in Figures 6.9 and 6.10 and think about how successful they are in fulfilling these aims. Be aware that they have been included purely for purposes of illustrating poster design and it is not intended that the text will be legible.

Make your poster eye-catching

A bright poster with an intriguing illustration will attract viewers to your poster. The poster in Figures 6.9 and 6.10 each have such an illustration; one is of a rat that appears to be under water but not at all distressed, and the other is of someone wearing a weird-looking contraption on their head. Both posters are colourful and have other illustrations and a passer-by would be drawn in to find out more.

Making the poster easy to navigate

Having attracted a viewer to the poster, he or she needs guidance to follow it in a logical manner. The poster in Figure 6.9 uses numbered boxes. Figure 6.10 uses well-recognised headings in the various boxes, starting with the

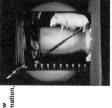
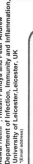
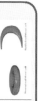
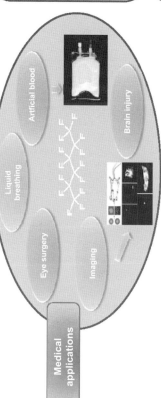

Figure 6.9 Student poster designed for a scientific but non-specialist audience, prepared at an early stage in the project. The viewer would be attracted to learn more by talking to the presenter. (Courtesy of Nawal Helmi, Peter Andrew, and Hitesh Pandya.)

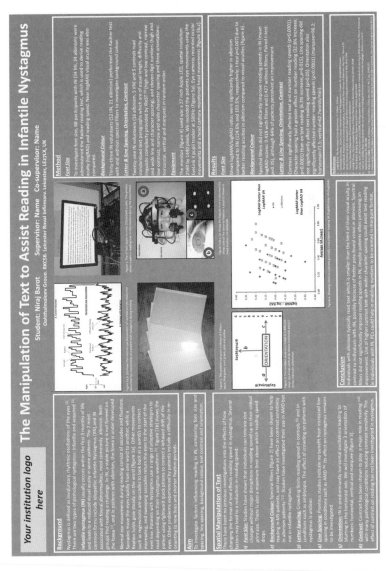

Figure 6.10 Student poster designed for staff and fellow students involved with an intercalated BSc. (Courtesy of Niraj Barot).

Background in the top left corner and working down the columns. The final box (Conclusion) is somewhat misplaced but the overall effect is pleasing.

Making the poster easy to read

The poster in Figure 6.9 contains little text, and the presenter has made good use of bullet points. This poster will be easy to read, even when the viewer is some distance away. The poster in Figure 6.10 has much more text, but therefore conveys more detailed information. In each example, the decision about how much text to include has been based on the audiences for which the posters have been prepared. The amount of text on Figure 6.10 limits the maximum font size that can be used, and the viewer will need to be fairly close to this poster to read it comfortably, particularly the legends to the figures. When designing your poster, think about how easy it will be to read the text. Be as economical as you can with the text, using bullet points rather than long sentences. Within reason, choose the largest font size you can. Choose a simple font, such as Arial, and differentiate headings and subheadings clearly from body text. This can be done by use of colour, font style, font size or a combination. Colour choices are a matter of personal preference but there should be a reasonable contrast between the colour of the background and the text. Look at examples of posters you may find on the walls of your department and see what combinations work well. Figures 6.9 and 6.10 both used white text on a mid-blue background, which is a common and effective combination. The text and background colours should not clash in a way that demands the use of sunglasses, but should serve to make the poster easy to read. Remember that red-green colour blindness is reasonably common and such a combination is best avoided.

Talking to your audience

Depending on the circumstances of your poster presentation, you may feel more or less self-conscious about standing around, waiting to talk about your work to those who have come to view it. Self-consciousness may lead you to want to shrink away from the poster stand, but resist this! You are in the game of promoting your work, after all! Stand so that it is obvious that you have ownership of the poster, but not in such a way as to obscure your prize illustration or the title. As viewers approach, you might like to greet them by saying something like, 'Hello. Would you like me to talk you through the poster?' If you get into a deep discussion, try to ensure – as far as possible – that you are not standing in a place that makes it impossible for others passing by to view your poster. If you do not know the person who has come to speak to you, take the opportunity to ask who they are and what their interest is, because this is a good opportunity to network. At the conclusion of the discussion, thank them for their interest and comments, and exchange contact details if necessary.

Making your own opportunities

There can be a few research projects where the students are not required to do either a presentation or a poster, and some institutions may require you to do both. If you can present your poster or give a presentation to another group of people, your work will be getting more exposure and the overall impact will increase. You will also get more feedback on the work, which could improve your project if it happens at an early stage, and the chance to network. Networking, or linking in with different individuals, will widen the range of people you can ask for help and advice. Promoting your work in this way will also strengthen your Curriculum Vitae.

What to do with your poster

If you have prepared a poster you will have to decide what to do with it afterwards. Your supervisor might have asked that it be pinned up on the wall outside the laboratory or in a corridor in the host department, and this is a frequent destination for posters. Others may adorn the wall of your bedroom until you come to move house, when suddenly it does not seem so vital any more. Although the posters may not have an infinite lifespan, because the science will be superseded, it is rather a pity if they get seen by only a very few people. Look around the buildings where you work and study, try and identify a suitable place, and ask if your poster can be displayed. You may want to involve other students in this so there is a display of several contrasting posters rather than just one. Do not restrict yourself to buildings occupied primarily by students and academic staff: there may be other venues where a poster could have more impact. A poster resulting from a project designed to look at links between physical fitness and blood cholesterol levels in young adults (mentioned in Chapter 2) could have maximum impact in the sports hall. By asking the Director of the Sports Hall if you can display the poster, you might open a discussion whereby he or she takes interest in the work and expresses a willingness to facilitate other projects in the future. (Even if this does not bring you direct benefit, your supervisor is likely to be extremely grateful). Joe's project (looking at whether medical and nursing students had a healthier diet than other students) from Chapter 4 might result in a poster that could be displayed in the student canteen, giving student something to consider as they queued to pay for their meals. Posters that have a simple health message might be ideally suited to be displayed in waiting rooms where they can be appreciated by patients and others. Do get permission before putting up posters in public areas, and think carefully about whether they are suitable. A poster with the title 'How Gentle Exercise Can Keep Your Heart Healthy' might be ideal for a cardiology outpatient clinic, but one entitled 'Audit of Cardiac Deaths in Hospital' in the same setting would not!

Where might you give a presentation?

Your supervisor might be the sort of person who actively encourages his or her students to attend meetings, submit articles for publication and give talks. If this is the case, you can follow their suggestions and guidance about where to go to raise your profile and that of the work. Do not be reticent about asking for opportunities, and ask colleagues and other students if they have any suggestions. It is likely that there are a range of opportunities where you could showcase what you have been doing. These could include attendance at national and societal meetings, for which you would probably have to submit an abstract that would be considered by a panel whose role is to decide which ones would go forward for a spoken presentation and which might be accepted for a poster presentation. Some societies have schemes to encourage students, such as a free registration for the student with the best abstract or much reduced registration costs. Look at relevant websites to see what meetings they are organising and see if you could submit your work. One factor in where you might go to attend a meeting is, of course, the cost. There will be the cost of registration and travel and possibly accommodation as well. Your supervisor should be honest about whether they have any funding to pay for you and may be able to suggest who you might approach to help cover your costs.

In addition to the subject specific conferences, there are conferences specifically for students. In the United Kingdom, the Royal Society of Medicine has a student section with opportunities to present research. One international meeting that has grown substantially since it began in 1993 is ISCOMS (International Student Congress of (bio)Medical Sciences), held each year in the Netherlands. This is a great opportunity to present your work to your peers from all over the world, either by spoken or poster presentation, which is relatively cheap to attend. If nobody from your institution has been to it before, why not get together with a group of your fellow project students and travel to ISCOMS?

Nearer to home, you may find various opportunities to speak about your work. Aside from any commitment that is a requirement of being a project student, you could offer to talk to different audiences. Speaking to various groups of people is likely to require you to prepare alternative talks – the outcome of your research is unaltered but how it is communicated may need changing.

Universities and colleges are keen to promote links with the communities in which they are based and, in particular, to encourage young people to consider higher education. You could enquire if there was some way you could link your project work with an institutional initiative, perhaps, by giving a talk to children at local schools. Speaking to a range of different audiences is terrific training and shows your willingness to engage with people other than your peers.

Consider Hannah's project in Chapter 4 (a review of pain relief in childbirth, including historical background and audit). If the midwives at her local hospital had regular meetings, they might be very glad to listen to what Hannah had researched. If your project has focused on a specific medical condition, there might be a patient support group who would be interested in your work. If you have had a bursary to support your project, offer to speak to the trustees who have supported you. Do not turn down opportunities to speak about your research, and take active steps to seek them out.

Other ways of raising profile and maximising impact

Occasionally, a project yields important results that are worthy of sharing with a wide audience, and you may want to issue a press release. Talk with your supervisor and get advice from the press officer of your institution before doing this because if the press get the wrong idea about something it could all end in tears. The idea of a press release is that the important message is expressed briefly and in a readily understandable form that can be easily propagated, and that there is a point of contact for anyone wanting more information. Usually any press release would be issued **after** the work had been published in peer-reviewed medical or scientific journals so that its credibility was established. Think back to Chapter 1 and imagine that Philip had worked on Dr White's project looking at reasons why patients sought medical advice following day case surgery. Imagine that he found that very many patients usually just needed reassurance, but were reticent about seeking medical advice. A draft press release is shown (Figure 6.11).

The press release can be picked up by any journalist who can then contact the originators and build up a story if he or she wants. Media local to the place where the release was issued are perhaps most likely to pick up the story, which could result in a radio interview if it was sufficiently interesting. The example above may not grab the media moguls, but someone researching patient satisfaction might just pick up on it and contact the researchers. When you have completed your project, try and write a press release as an exercise, and see how exciting and relevant you can make it appear.

Issued by the University of Anywhere Press office on 6 December 2011

'Send me home – but please check I'm OK'

Patients are happy to go home after day case surgery, but many of them are anxious about things the following day and would like a phone call from a nurse or other professional to check their recovery is progressing. This is the main finding of a research project done by medical student Philip Baxter and his supervisor Dr Charlotte White.

Philip explains what they did,' We interviewed patients who had had day case surgery and asked them all sorts of things about how they felt afterwards, and their overwhelming response was they were happy to be home, but many of them wanted reassurance the following day. Most of them took no action, but stayed at home feeling anxious. One of the patients hardly slept because she was worried about rolling onto her scar, but she said 'it seemed such a silly thing to make a special telephone call just for that'. Philip interviewed over 50 patients and found that 83% would have valued a phone call to check on their progress. The type of surgery was not important, and women and men were equally anxious.

Dr White says, 'Philip's study highlighted an aspect of patient satisfaction we had not appreciated at the GP practice. We had not realised how many of them are reluctant to call if they are worried. It is very important that our patients recognise that we care about their anxieties. As a result of Philip's study we now ensure that every patient having day-case surgery gets a phone call at home from one of the practice team so they have the opportunity to ask anything, however trivial it may seem'.

Publication: Baxter, P. and White, C. (2011) Patient anxiety after day-case surgery. Journal of Caring Medicine, 42,1706.

For more information contact:

Dr C White
HappyBunny GP Practice
Anywhere
Tel. 04562 878763 e: cwhite@happybunny.org

Figure 6.11 Format of a possible press release at the conclusion of the project.

Other contemporary ways of disseminating your research include publishing a blog. This could be one way of telling anyone with an interest what you were doing, and if you are an inveterate blogger you may want to do this. However, be extremely cautious, especially about disseminating any results, and talk to your supervisor in advance. You may find that you publish data that you then need to revise, or you make a fundamental mistake. Your supervisor may not want the output of their lab to be made available to any competitors. Although you may have done the work, you do not have sole rights over the data. Of course, using a blog or a Facebook page to tell all your mates about how hard you are working or how exciting you find your project is fine, but it is probably best to leave it at that.

Other ways of making an impact may be to use your skills and knowledge in a teaching capacity. This can be very diverse, including writing an improved patient information leaflet, or developing a teaching resource for other students. The student section of the website of the Society for General Microbiology includes a quiz for teenagers, which was developed as part of an undergraduate project. Be as creative as you can in finding ways of making your research project have a real impact; the personal benefits in terms of the whole research project experience will be enormously enhanced.

SUMMARY

Your research project will need to be written up as a dissertation, and you may also be required to give a spoken or a poster presentation. Think about how you might gain added advantage from your research project by presenting it outside your home institution.

Spoken presentations can be daunting but the key to a good presentation lies in preparation and practice. Avoid the common fault of trying to pack in too much information: a talk with a more modest amount of information that is clearly presented so everyone in the audience can understand the main points is much better than subjecting your audience to a barrage of complicated slides at breakneck speed.

Poster presentations at meetings will require that the presenter is present to discuss the work with viewers, but a good, eye-catching poster can continue in a 'standalone' context, so why not try and find a prestigious final location for your work?

Be creative about getting your research publicised through press releases and social media, but be aware that this must only be done with support and approval of your supervisor.

Chapter 7 **Preparing for your assessment**

CHAPTER OVERVIEW

Although students do not usually have any control over the method by which their research project is assessed, there are several things that can be done to enhance the chances of doing well. This chapter emphasises the need for the student to familiarise themselves with the method of assessment, distribution of marks and any guidance provided to the examiners. Where there is to be a *viva voce* examination, there is much that can be done to prepare for this, and the chapter emphasises the importance of the practice viva. Some tips are given on final preparations. Finally, the issue of what to do when deadlines or other requirements cannot be met is addressed.

You may have started to prepare for your assessment before you began your project. You probably knew something about the method of assessment at the outset, particularly if it includes a viva or spoken examination. Consciously or subconsciously, your choice of topic may have been influenced by whether you thought it was one that could be readily packaged into something likely to rate highly in an assessment. Even if you had no choice in the topic of your research, you may have steered your work into something that the examiners are likely to look upon with favour! Whether you considered your assessment at the early stages or not, it pays to prepare yourself well in advance. Remember the five 'Ps' – proper preparation prevents poor performance. Even though you may not know what will most impress the examiners, you can put yourself in a position to achieve good marks with a bit of forethought and preparation.

How to do your Research Project: A Guide for Students in Medicine and the Health Sciences, First Edition. Caroline Beardsmore.
© 2013 John Wiley & Sons, Ltd. Published 2013 by John Wiley & Sons, Ltd.

Find out about how the work is assessed

It is essential to know how your work is going to be assessed if you are to do well. Details should be readily available from your project handbook, website or similar. The important things to focus on are how marks are distributed, the people who are involved in assessment and what guidance they may be given about marking.

Distribution of marks

Some institutions may work with a system of numerical marks, whereas others may provide guidance for examiners on assigning a grade or degree classification. Whichever system is used, you should have access to how your institution assesses your project. The distribution of marks will vary from one institution to another, but may include marks for the written dissertation and for a viva or spoken presentation. You should find out at an early stage how your work is to be evaluated so that you can best prepare for each aspect of your assessment. The marking system as it relates to your dissertation is likely to include separate components for scientific content and presentation. Make sure you are familiar with this, so that you can 'cover all bases' in your written work (see Chapter 5). It is worth reiterating the importance of following any guidance or instructions to the letter. For example, writing a report that substantially exceeds the word count will not impress the examiners with the extent of your knowledge but is more likely to irritate them because you have not followed the instructions and they have to spend extra time reading your work.

Aside from the dissertation, marks may be awarded for a spoken presentation and/or a viva, or possibly some other type of presentation such as a poster. If these form a part of your assessment, you need to allocate sufficient preparation time so that you perform to the best of your ability.

Input from your supervisor

Some institutions include the supervisor as one of your examiners because he or she will have observed your skills and performance. Others may **not** include the supervisor as an examiner to avoid any possible suggestion of bias. In these cases, the supervisor may be asked to provide a report for the examiners on the laboratory performance of the student. The supervisor is usually the best person to assess how good the student has been at the practical aspects of the work. With a laboratory project, this covers their practical skills and techniques. A project involving work with human subjects will inevitably require good interpersonal skills. Good organisation is essential for a library or a data-handling project. Whether or not your supervisor is also one of your examiners, you should ensure that your laboratory work is carried out according to the best laboratory practice, and seen to be so (see Chapter 2). If you are unsure about exactly how things should be done, then it is important to ask at an early stage. Once your project is under way, you might want to check with your supervisor if they are satisfied with this aspect of your work, or if there is a room for improvement.

Internal and external examiners

Other examiners will include external and internal examiners. The internal examiners will be staff members from your own institution and, unless they are newly appointed to their posts, they will be familiar with the type of assessment they will be undertaking. All examiners will be provided with the guidelines they need to assess the projects fairly and consistently. As in most summative assessments, there will usually be double marking and/or moderating. These ensure that the assessments are as fair and transparent as it is possible to make them. Where work is double marked, the two markers will work independently and each will assign marks or a grade. Usually the two sets of marks or grades are averaged but, if they differ by a substantial amount, a third person or a moderator may be involved to help decide the appropriate mark for the project. Moderators will frequently have a role in ensuring consistency 'across the board'. Even with clear guidelines about how to assign a grade or degree classification to a piece of work, some individual assessors will tend to mark more strictly than others, which is particularly relevant for projects that fall on a borderline. One examiner might consider a project to be excellent in some respects but average in others and would assign a degree classification of upper second-class honours (a 2.1 degree), but another examiner looking at the same project might think that, overall, the standard was so good that first-class honours should be awarded. This is where moderation comes in to play.

Specific responsibilities of external examiners

The role of an external examiner has much in common with that of a moderator. External examiners are senior staff from other institutions directly involved in teaching and examining in the same or very closely related subjects. The system of external examiners has been developed to provide consistency of standards between different institutions, so that a degree from one college or university is equivalent to that from another. The perspective of an external examiner is valuable because he or she can comment on all aspects of the course and make recommendations for improvements and changes. It is likely that staff members from your own institution also act as external examiners elsewhere and glean ideas from other institutions. This should not be seen as stealing other people's good ideas, but rather as a means of sharing the best academic practice. The external examiner is likely to spend time at your college or university at examination time and share in the assessment process, especially where it involves a viva or spoken component. The external examiner may ask to see as many of the pieces of assessed work as he or she likes and to participate in whichever vivas he or she wants. Typically, the external examiner will ask to see a subset of projects in order to get an overview of the whole cohort of students and projects. For example, in a cohort of 50 students, the external examiner might ask to see the top five projects, five projects judged to be typical or middle-ranking, and the weakest five projects. He or she may also want to see those judged to be on the borderlines of degree classifications and any where there were particular extenuating circumstances for the student.

Anonymity of marking

Projects may be marked anonymously, so that the markers do not know which student has produced the work they are assessing. Even if this is the case, internal examiners may know – or guess – the supervisor and have some idea about which student's work they are looking at. This should not influence their marking in any way. In other places the examiners will know the student whose work they are assessing. Whether or not the examiners know the student, they should be acting impartially at all stages.

Any underhand attempts to influence the outcome of your assessment would constitute a serious disciplinary offence. Do not even consider it! Having said that, you can present your work in the best possible way to gain a high mark. For example, if you know that one of the examiners is an expert in Health Economics, you may be prompted to include some discussion on the financial aspects of the topic you have been working on. If your examiners include a pharmacologist or a developmental expert, have you considered which common drugs or medications should be mentioned in your dissertation, or if your research is relevant for a particular developmental stage or time of life? While any project may have many facets, knowing the areas of expertise of your examiners may prompt you to consider one you previously had not thought about.

Role of the exam board

Once the examiners have done their work, an exam board will usually consider and approve their recommendations. This higher level of scrutiny is an additional mechanism for moderation, should it prove needed. Even with the best guidelines and regulations, there is always the chance of unexpected events at each stage of any course, including the assessment, and an exam board can consider how best to manage such unforeseen circumstances.

Guidance given to examiners regarding the dissertation

Guidance given to examiners is likely to be available to students, and this may be helpful as you prepare, both for handing in your dissertation and getting ready for a viva. If you put yourself in the examiner's position, and know what he or she is looking for, you are more likely to be able to deliver what they are looking for. This may be particularly relevant if they are recommending a degree classification. Table 7.1 is an example of what examiners may be looking for in a dissertation, so you can see how well your own work measures up!

Preparing for a viva examination (having a practice viva)

Other than your written dissertation, your assessment may also include spoken or poster presentations, which are covered in Chapter 6. Another form of assessment is the viva exam. 'Viva' is short for '*viva voce*', the Latin phrase that means 'the living voice' – in other words, a spoken examination. The purpose of the viva is to give the examiners an opportunity to explore the depth of your understanding of the topic and assess how well you can defend your work and see it in a wider context.

Practise talking about your project

Although the precise questions you may be asked cannot be known in advance you can prepare yourself for your viva, so that the outcome is the best you can make it. A practice viva is invaluable, so if your supervisor does not arrange this for you, find somebody who will act as an examiner. Ideally, this would be someone with some background knowledge of the area you have been working in, but this is not essential because the key thing is for you to talk about your work to another person. It is vital that you are able to communicate what you have been doing to other people. It is likely that you have been asked, in social settings, what you are doing and each opportunity should be seen as a chance to explain your work. The detail into which you go will depend on the situation but you should be able to provide a satisfactory answer to anyone who asks. Think about Emma's project in Chapter 5, with the possible title 'Factors influencing Thingummy Receptor Density in Airway Smooth Muscle', and consider what she might say to someone who asked her what the project was about. To someone who had no background knowledge in science or medicine, she might say, 'People with asthma have airways – the breathing tubes – that are very sensitive and these readily narrow down. This can be caused by the muscles in the airways which, when they shorten,

Table 7.1 Example of what examiners might be looking for in a dissertation

Formulation of the research question	Is the research question precisely formulated and clearly expressed? Is it justified, perhaps, by identifying a gap in the literature?
Ethics	If there was any requirement for permission from a Research Ethics Committee, is the approval clearly documented?
Introduction and background	This should be relevant and presented in a logical manner, should refer to all the major relevant research papers and be up to date.
Choice of methodology	The choice of methods should be appropriate to answer the question(s) posed.
Description of methods	Is the description of the methods sufficiently detailed, including description of the methods of analysis (choice of statistical tests) if appropriate?
Results	Results should be clearly presented in a format suitable to the data. The analysis should be transparent. Where appropriate, appendices can be used to make data available that is not suitable for presentation in the main text.
Discussion	Findings should be summarised, interpreted and put into context. Conclusions should be supported by the evidence presented.
Referencing	This should be accurate and presented in a recognised format.
Presentation	The dissertation should be easy to navigate, with numbered pages, and headings and subheadings that are logical. Illustrations, figures and tables should be easy to understand, with titles, legends and footnotes that guide the reader. Grammar and spelling should be of a high standard.
Originality and critical thinking	Critical thinking and insight should be evident throughout the dissertation, and originality should be demonstrated where appropriate.

cause the airways to constrict. The muscle cells have receptors on the surface that respond to certain compounds in the surrounding fluid, influencing what the muscles do. My project looks at the density of these receptors – how many there are on each cell – and some of the things that affect this.' This simple explanation contains no scientific jargon and can stand alone. If the questioner wants to ask more details then he or she has not been put off by specialist language. In contrast, when talking to a fellow student taking a similar course of study, Emma would probably use more technical language, introducing terms such as 'bronchoconstriction' and 'agonist'. The key to describing your project is to start with a straightforward, broad-brush approach before moving on to the finer details, whoever is asking the questions. Practise talking about your project whenever you can. The more opportunity you have to talk about your work, the better you become at it.

The general questions

A mock viva, however, is best if your 'examiner' is able to go into some depth in the questioning. It is not essential that they read every page of your dissertation, but if they have some time to look at it in advance they will be able to prepare some more searching questions. In thinking about your viva – or your mock viva – you may be able to predict some of the questions that are likely to come up. Some of these are likely to be general questions, designed to allow you free rein to talk about your work, or to help you relax at the start of the viva. Examples are shown (Box 7.1), and you should be able to answer any of these if asked.

Box 7.1   General questions that may be asked at a viva examination

---

Tell us, in a few sentences, what your project was all about.
What was the most challenging thing you faced in your project?
Why did you choose this particular topic for your research project?
Your research project relates to (*name of condition or disease*). Tell us a bit more about it – how common is it, for example?
What would you say was the most important finding of your research project?
If you could start the project all over again, is there anything that you would do differently? If you were continuing with this project, what would you do next?
What did you enjoy most about your research project?

Being able to answer the general questions will usually get the viva off to a good start. You may be uncertain how long the examiners expect you to speak for, but open questions such as these usually invite something more than just a few words. Your answer to question 2, for example, might be that 'Performing the assay for compound X was the most difficult part of the project...', but if you can add something like '... so I asked one of the technicians to show me exactly what she did, and then when I had learned some helpful tips it seemed to go much more smoothly'. The more complete answer, showing that you had some initiative, gives a more positive impression than the first part on its own. Your answer to question 3 might be 'I chose this topic because I have always been interested in diabetes', but expanding on this to say 'because the potential consequences of diabetes are so wide ranging, and it is a condition that is becoming increasingly common in our society' is a more satisfactory response. Do beware of trying to say too much, however, and giving the examiners a lecture on diabetes! If you are not sure, you can pause and ask them if they would like you to say more. This gives them the chance to move on if they are ready.

The difficult questions

You will probably know which part of your research project is likely to give rise to difficult questions, so you should prepare your answers for these. Do not dismiss the areas of weakness, but acknowledge the limitations of your work while at the same time trying to appear positive. Think about Joe's project in Chapter 5, comparing the diets of different groups of students. He might have found that the response rate of the students was poor, so that he did not get as many questionnaires returned as he would have liked. When being questioned about this, he might say, 'The response rate was too small for my findings to show much of statistical significance, and if I had been able to extend the study time for another 3 months I might have been able to improve on this. Nevertheless, there was a strong trend that suggested (*something*), and this was clearly supported by the qualitative findings.' Joe is not making excuses, but rather providing a suggestion for improving the work and shifting the discussion to something he would like the questioner to focus on!

Finally in preparing for your viva or your mock viva, check through the illustrations and diagrams. You may be asked to explain or expand on one of these. It is so easy to access and use a diagram from an external source, with permission, but can you fully explain what it shows? Does it contain abbreviations that you are unfamiliar with? Preparing your own diagrams may take longer but you will be sure to understand them when they are complete!

When your mock viva or vivas are complete, ask your 'examiners' for feedback on your performance and for advice on anything you could improve on. This may be repeated use of certain words or phrases, minor habits such as twisting your hands together or failing to make eye contact when being asked a question. These may be small matters, but they can all help you give a confident and competent performance on the day.

Final preparations, calming nerves and getting into a good frame of mind

Even when your mock vivas have given you plenty of practice at talking about your research and the confidence that you can answer questions on all aspects of the project, there are still some things you can do ahead of time so that you are properly prepared. The day before your viva, make sure you have your own copy of your dissertation and anything else you plan to take with you all ready and in your bag. Other things could include your laboratory book, which might be a requirement, copies of key references and perhaps a small piece of equipment or an example of raw data that could not be included in your dissertation. If appropriate, take a laptop with a short video clip of an aspect of your experimental work. (If you do this, do not assume your examiners will want to watch it. A project in which ciliary beat frequency was measured using high-resolution video imaging may pique their interest, but a sequence showing how you pipetted a solution into a test tube is boring and adds nothing to your assessment!) Your bag may also contain a bottle of water, in case this is not provided at the viva, and a pack of tissues. On the front of your dissertation, put a post-it note to yourself saying 'TURN OFF MOBILE PHONE', so that when you go in for the viva you will be prompted to do this if it was something you might otherwise have overlooked.

In addition to preparing your bag, make sure you know exactly where your viva is to be held and if it is in an unfamiliar room or building make sure you know how to get there. Where will you sit and wait if you are there ahead of time, or if the examiners are late in calling you in? Do you know where the nearest loo is located? If you are arriving by a car or a bike, will you be able to park at that time of day, and is there somewhere to secure your bicycle?

Students frequently ask how they should dress, and specifically if they should wear a suit for a viva. It is unlikely that there are institutional guidelines about such matters. Whatever you decide to wear, it is important that you feel comfortable in what you are wearing while, at the same time, showing that you recognise the importance of the viva by being reasonably smart. Of course you are not being marked on what you are wearing, but do not let your attire give your examiners any cause to comment, even if only inwardly! Get your clothes ready the day before, so that you can check that there are no unfortunate stains, missing buttons and so on.

It is likely that you will know several other students in the same situation as yourself. Some individuals convey a sense of calm confidence whereas others seem to generate high levels of stress in everyone around them. Where you have a choice, spend time in the company of the former and avoid the latter! You are preparing for your own assessment and not acting as an agony aunt for everyone else.

Although you may be apprehensive, try to get a good sleep the night before your viva. At that time there is little more you can do to prepare yourself and if you are well rested you are likely to perform better. Do not skip breakfast. Even if you do not feel like it, have something to eat so that you do not risk feeling faint at viva time. All students are likely to be apprehensive or anxious or may be very nervous depending on their personalities. If you are the type of person who gets wound up under pressure, try to find things to do that will help to calm your nerves and take your mind off the viva during the previous 24 hours. This might include going for a walk, a swim, watching a film or relaxing in a deep bath. Avoid excessive alcohol or stimulants. Reassure yourself that you have worked hard, that you are the expert on your own project and that you will be able to talk about it enthusiastically at your viva. Picture yourself at your viva, performing competently and walking out afterwards having given the best account of your research project. Keep that picture in mind and maintain a positive attitude. Your viva will probably fly past and you will come out wondering why you ever got nervous in the first place.

After your viva

Some institutions maintain the practice of telling the students the outcome of the assessment shortly after the viva. The examiners confer, reach their decision and then meet again with the student to tell them their recommendation and give feedback. If you receive the result in this manner it may be difficult to respond because you may not be able to anticipate the outcome. If you are disappointed, then it is likely that the examiners will give you some guidance as to the areas of weakness and you should try to take note of their comments. When you have had some time to reflect and discuss things with your supervisor, your disappointment may lessen. In the unlikely event that you feel the outcome is grossly unfair, take some time to think things through and discuss matters with an appropriate member of staff before launching into potential complaints (see Chapter 8). It is much more usual for students to be satisfied with a good result, in which case it would be appropriate simply to thank the examiners. Your supervisor, and possibly others who have supported you through your project, will also be keen to find out how your viva went, so do not neglect to tell them the outcome. The chances are that they will be joining you in celebrations!

What happens if you cannot meet your assessment deadlines or requirements?

Sometimes students have extenuating circumstances that need to be taken into account for the purposes of their assessment. This umbrella term covers things that crop up unexpectedly that might affect your work and that should reasonably be taken into account in your assessment, or might be grounds for an extension to the date of submission. On any course, there is always the possibility that a student may have a significant health problem or suffer bereavement of a close family member and your institution will be sympathetic. Exactly how such matters are handled will vary, but in most cases a pragmatic approach will be adopted. A student who sprains his or her wrist early in the course of their project and cannot type may well be able to continue to make progress in other ways and not need an extension, whereas the same injury close to the date of completion, when the student is busy writing their dissertation, may be grounds for an extension. In this example, an alternative approach to the assessment might be for the student to submit their written work to date and have an extended viva examination to cover the aspects that had not been committed to paper.

When the extenuating circumstances involve your health, it is likely that you will be asked for evidence of this, such as a letter from your doctor or other health professional. If you feel that your circumstances warrant some form of special treatment or dispensation, do speak to your supervisor about this. If they do not know the full circumstances, they may not be in a position to advise you or to act as your advocate. It is possible that any request for extenuating circumstances needs to come through the supervisor in any case. If you cannot speak to your supervisor (for whatever reason) then speak to your mentor, course convenor or a staff member in whom you can confide, so that you get the advice and support you may need. If your problem is deeply personal, then you can ask that the precise details be kept confidential, or only made available to those people who need to know.

Sometimes things happen that are unrelated to health or personal circumstances and could not have been foreseen. It is not unknown for supervisors to fall ill, move to another institution, or be suspended from their work in the course of a student project. If this happens then you need to make sure that the effect (real or potential) is flagged up with your course convenor at an early stage. The duration of some problems may be impossible to predict, so it is better to plan for the worst and hope for the best than to just keep your fingers crossed! When the difficulty is something that affects any laboratory or practical work you may be doing then there may be an opportunity to refocus your project. For example, a student whose project involved perfusion experiments on pig kidneys had a major disruption when foot-and-mouth disease caused the closure of the nation's abattoirs. Under these circumstances, the project was modified so that he could use histological slides to continue research in the same area of interest. It was not the work as originally envisaged, but he still had a good project with an excellent outcome.

Not all requests for extensions to your hand-in date, or other forms of dispensation, will necessarily be granted. Blaming the library for taking a few days to get an essential reprint or complaining that the print room needs 48 hours notice to print and bind your dissertation are not likely to be viewed sympathetically.

Sometimes students will try and soldier on with their work against a background of huge personal or family problems, thinking that admitting they are under pressure will be seen as a sign of weakness. It is far better to be honest about such things with your supervisor who can then make allowances (if appropriate) and may be able to suggest sources of advice and support. Most supervisors (unless they are very new to their post) will have worked with students whose lives have been going through a time of turbulence and will show understanding. If you are hesitant about speaking to your supervisor, identify another staff member that you find approachable and speak to him or her. Staff who keep a box of tissues on their office desks are often the ones to whom students will gravitate at times of stress! What is important is that if you are experiencing difficulties, you bring these to the attention of someone responsible for the course or the module at an early stage.

SUMMARY

Know exactly how your work is to be assessed and how marks are to be distributed. Make sure that your written work clearly meets the requirements that the examiners will be looking for.

If you are to have a viva voce exam, take every opportunity to talk about your project. Make sure you have at least one practice viva. Think about the likely questions and prepare your responses. Make sure you are fully prepared for your viva the day before it is scheduled; that way you can focus on keeping calm and relaxed beforehand. Avoid people who are likely to make you feel stressed.

If there are reasons why you may fail to meet a deadline or other requirement of your course, make sure that someone with responsibility for you or your project is aware of this at the earliest opportunity.

Chapter 8 **When things go wrong**

CHAPTER OVERVIEW

Research projects are challenging and few of them run without any problems whatsoever. In many cases these are readily addressed and the progress is smooth, but more serious matters can arise at any stage. This chapter discusses some of the problems that might arise with the project itself and how these might be addressed. Difficulties that can arise with supervision are covered, including those where there is a breakdown in communication, which may lead to simple misunderstandings. The problems that students face that are unrelated to their research, but affect their work, are discussed in some detail. The overarching message of this chapter is the importance of addressing problems at an early stage and not 'soldiering on' in the hope that they will disappear. Finally problems of a procedural nature, particularly relating to assessment, are covered.

If you think things are not going well, or if you have any problems, do not ignore them. It is much better to sort out a small problem early than wait until it is a big problem. By then, there is less time for any sorting-out to be done. In any problem solving, your supervisor should be your main source of support, but occasionally he or she cannot see what you are struggling with, or they might be the source of the problem! If your supervisor is not available or is part of the problem, as you perceive it, remember that most institutions will have other processes to help students with difficulties (personal tutors, course convenors, student counselling services), and these are in place for a purpose. It is up to you to decide if you are encountering problems that warrant seeking help or advice, but you should never be afraid to ask. Your research project is

How to do your Research Project: A Guide for Students in Medicine and the Health Sciences,
First Edition. Caroline Beardsmore.
© 2013 John Wiley & Sons, Ltd. Published 2013 by John Wiley & Sons, Ltd.

likely to be the first one you have ever done; for the staff it is probably one of many and they can best judge if you are worrying unnecessarily and provide reassurance or, alternatively, if action needs to be taken.

What sort of problems might I encounter?

Very few research projects are completed without any problems at all, unless they are extremely straightforward and of short duration. The problems encountered in research projects will range from the trivial to the almost catastrophic and from the predictable to those that could never have been envisaged. Although each project is unique, the problems experienced by students may not be novel and you should be able to access help to cope with all eventualities. Most problems can be divided into one of three categories: those relating to the project, the supervisor or the student. A smaller category will be procedural problems that may occasionally occur.

Problems with the project

The range of problems you might encounter is as varied as the projects themselves, but some of the commoner ones are detailed below.

Poor recruitment

A common problem with many projects is that the number of subjects recruited or measurements made falls short of that which was anticipated. This may mean that the statistical power of the project is insufficient to answer the questions posed. This may not jeopardise your marks or grades, since you are likely to be assessed on your dissertation, skills, approach, abilities and so on and not solely on your results. However, it is disappointing for all concerned. Reasons for poor recruitment of people (whether patients or other volunteers) are many, and you should try and identify these – preferably before you start! If your supervisor has supervised projects along similar lines before, then there is a very good chance that he or she will have a good idea of the likely recruitment rates for what you are going to do. If you are doing something rather more novel, then almost certainly the recruitment strategy will have been approved by the Research Ethics Committee. If you find that the recruitment is going badly, then you need to identify the reasons for this as soon as possible, and try to ask other people if they can suggest how you can improve your recruitment. If you do fall behind with other things (such as the literature searching or your writing tasks), there may be the possibility of catch-up by doing more work in the evenings or at weekends, but it is much more difficult to catch up with recruitment, hence the need for rapid action.

One of the keys to success in recruiting people, whether patients or healthy volunteers, is the effectiveness of a personal approach. You may have a leaflet that gives all the essential information about your project but, if left on a counter or worktop, it can be easily ignored or overlooked. If you approach someone with a friendly greeting, say something like 'I wonder if I can ask you to read through this leaflet and think whether you might be able to contribute to the project? If you'd like to speak to me after you have read it, I'll be at the desk until the end of clinic', your success rate will increase. Personal approaches win hands down, every time.

If people decline to take part in your project, and if it is appropriate to do so, you might ask them if they are prepared to tell you why they declined. Even if the information does not help you to improve the recruitment rate, it could serve to explain in your dissertation why the target was not reached.

Sometimes poor recruitment can be addressed by widening the eligibility criteria for the project, for example, by lowering the minimum age for participation or increasing the upper limit of body mass index for participation. Do remember that changes in your recruitment strategy or eligibility criteria are likely to require an amendment to any Research Ethics Committee approval.

Finding your project is not unique

Occasionally, a student might find that they are working on a project that seems to have a lot in common with that of another student based in the same laboratory or workplace setting. The student – rightly – might be concerned that the uniqueness of his or her own project is in doubt, since research written up and submitted as part of a university degree is expected to be unique. The student might worry about the possible accusations of plagiarism. If you are in this situation, you should speak to your supervisor and ask what part of the work (assuming you are part of a team) can be clearly identified as yours. In most cases this should be straightforward. There are occasions when, quite legitimately, you are duplicating someone else's work. This may be to confirm that you can replicate their techniques before extending into something that is more properly your own.

From time to time, someone working on a research project can find out that another group publishes a paper or an abstract that duplicates the work they are doing. It can be maddening to find that someone else 'got there first' but, if it happens to you, this is most unlikely to invalidate your work. Your project does not dictate that you should publish anything and your marks should be unaffected. What you will need to do is compare your work with the newly published item and highlight any differences, whether in methodology, results or interpretation.

Breakdown of essential equipment

If your project requires a piece of equipment that breaks or malfunctions while you are using it, then no doubt you will try to see what the problem is and try to fix it. Your next step is likely to be asking a more experienced user if they can help. If this is the case, try to observe the repair so that you can do it yourself the next time. If the equipment cannot be repaired more or less on the spot, then you should report the breakdown to your supervisor and/or laboratory manager, and ask the likely timescale for the repair. If the equipment broke down when you were setting it up or using it, you may need to explain what you were doing and exactly what happened. If the equipment was linked to any form of computer, make a precise note of any error messages as this may assist with diagnosing the problem. Put a notice on the equipment to state that it is broken and alert others who may be preparing to use it, so they do not waste time or experimental material unnecessarily.

If the timescale for the repair is short enough that it will not have a major impact on your work then there may not be much else to be done. However, the interruption to your work will be lessened if you can borrow equipment from another laboratory, so try asking your supervisor if he or she can suggest where else you might go to continue practical work. Aside from the obvious benefit of being able to continue your work, you may make new contacts with whom to discuss your work and its implications.

Some projects are dependent on specific pieces of equipment, and if these are expensive to purchase and maintain there may not be a backup if they break down. Such pieces of equipment are likely to be used by other individuals and groups and may be under a maintenance contract, so that if they break down someone from the manufacturing company or an agent will come and repair them within a set time period. In these circumstances, you are likely to be one of several people waiting for the repair and the laboratory manager or your supervisor can let you know the timescales. If you are part of a small group, you may be able to help by liaising with the manufacturer over the repair, for example, by running a test on the equipment and reporting the outcome. Getting involved with this will help you to learn more about the equipment you are using, and may put you at the front of the queue when the equipment is repaired!

Occasionally your practical work may have a major hold-up due to equipment failure. A delay of a few days is not likely to be critical, but one of several weeks most certainly will. Discuss with your supervisor at an early stage what you might do to overcome the delay and explore where you might go to find an alternative. If you are based in a hospital laboratory, perhaps a university laboratory may be able to help out – and vice versa. Some examples are shown in the textbox below. If, however, the delay is unavoidable (and possibly open-ended) then it would be judicious to discuss whether the project could be reorientated to allow you to place more emphasis on a different aspect. If you can be reasonably certain about when your equipment will be fully functional once more, you will be able to spend time on other aspects of your project (perhaps the reading and writing parts) while the practical work is put 'on hold'. Whatever you do, do not waste precious time waiting for something to be repaired.

In many cases, the disruptions caused by equipment breakdown do not have a major impact on the project and are just a part of daily life in research. As such, they may not merit a mention in your dissertation. If you have had your work severely hampered or curtailed by equipment breakdown then you may not want this to be overlooked. It may be appropriate to include a section in your dissertation or project write-up that addresses practical limitations to the project. This will give you an opportunity to explain the specific problems you faced, and state what you did to overcome these, so that the assessors or examiners can be aware of the challenges to your work.

Alex's project was based on a kidney perfusion model and required him to collect a fresh bovine kidney from the local abattoir on a weekly basis. He anticipated using eight kidneys, but after week 4 he was told that the abattoir was to be unexpectedly closed for an indeterminate period.

Alex's first response might be to find out which other abattoirs were located within a reasonable distance of his place of work. With luck, there may be another potential source of supply. This might necessitate his travelling some distance to fetch the kidneys, possibly requiring a taxi if he did not have his own transport and needed to get the kidneys to the laboratory within a short time after removal. He (or his supervisor) might need to visit the new abattoir to discuss their requirements precisely, especially, if it was not used to supplying research institutions. The personal approach may well be needed to establish a good working relationship and there may be a delay in restarting the experimental work so that Alex might not achieve his target of eight kidneys.

In parallel with this approach, Alex could approach the animal house within his own institution to find out if there was any possibility of acquiring mammalian kidneys from a different species that he could use in his experimental work. Of course, inter-species differences would mean that data could not be combined, but Alex could build in some comparative physiology into his project and turn an unfortunate situation into an advantage.

Devender relied on mass spectroscopy to measure volatile organic compounds in samples of exhaled breath. She had a message one day from the technician who was helping her to say that the machine had broken down. The technician was going on leave the following day and had arranged for the repairman to come 3 weeks later so that he was present at the time of the repair, 'because whenever they fix one thing they always mess up something else if you don't stand over them'.

Devender's first action would be to speak in person to the technician and ask if the repair could be brought forward, as the delay would hold up her project substantially. She would offer to be present for the duration of the time that the repairman was working on the machine, take full notes of what was done, and run any tests or calibrations the technician suggested. With luck, her offer of 'supervising' the repair would be accepted and she would soon be working again. In the bargain, she might also learn a lot about the equipment she was so reliant on.

Lauren used cell culture facilities extensively in her project. As she approached the midpoint of her practical work, there were several cases of infected cultures and the cell culture facility was closed until it had been thoroughly cleaned and all equipment sterilised. There was no date given for when it was likely to reopen.

This would be a major problem for Lauren, and one that she would need to discuss with her supervisor. Since she would not be the only person affected, she should ask the others if they had contingency plans, thereby finding out if there were alternative facilities she might use. In most universities there will be more than one department with cell culture facilities so, in consultation with her supervisor, she could contact other departments or research groups to see if she could continue her work elsewhere. She might need to undergo additional local training, since anyone in charge of a cell culture facility is unlikely to welcome 'refugees' from an infected facility without first being sure they can work within standard procedures. Whether or not she is able to continue her work elsewhere, Lauren should ask her supervisor if there is some way that her project might be extended without the need for cell culture. The time frame of her project would be relevant here, and it might be more sensible for her to use the time writing an extended review, for example.

Problems with the supervisor

Supervisors are only human and may themselves be facing some of the same challenges as their students, including personal, financial or professional difficulties. If your supervisor is ill or bereaved, then they will be away from work and unavailable to support you on a day-to-day basis or have discussions about what you should be doing. Unless you are part of a very small group or if the absence is of a long duration, it is likely that others can help and your progress will not be significantly affected. Even if your supervisor is absent, he or she may be in touch by e-mail to provide you with direction. If it becomes obvious that your supervisor will not be able to provide the input that was originally envisaged, then seek advice from someone with the responsibility for the student research projects, or the head of the department in which you are working. They may already be aware of your circumstances, but this may not be the case, particularly, in a large institution where students are spread in different departments and across several sites. In most cases, it should be possible to identify someone (or more than one person) who can step in to ensure your project runs as smoothly as possible. The absence of the supervisor might, on occasion, lead to some inevitable modification of your project, so try to see it as an opportunity to do something different, rather than an obstacle to your progress.

The timing of when a supervisor may become unavailable can influence what happens to the students. If, very early in the project, it is clear that the supervisor will require a long absence, then it might be best for the student to change to a different project and supervisor. If you have put a lot of effort into selecting the area in which you want to work, and helping to design your project, this will be frustrating but you will be able to understand that it is likely to be your best option. If your project is well advanced when your supervisor needs a leave of absence, then others will be able to advise you on writing your dissertation, which may not necessarily require a detailed knowledge of your subject matter.

Occasionally a supervisor will take up a new job at a different institution during the time when they are supervising research project students. You may feel let down if you planned your project with this supervisor, joined their team, then 5 minutes later they tell you that they are moving somewhere else! The reason, of course, is that nobody advertises the fact that they are applying for a new job in case they are not appointed! They will generally continue to work without interruption even when applying or being considered for another job.

The timescale for academic staff to resign from one post and begin another is usually one term, so a supervisor will not disappear overnight. Only if your project extends beyond the date when your supervisor leaves are you likely to be affected. In many cases when someone leaves, they will be given an honorary contract with their original institution, to allow them to complete their supervisory responsibilities, so you may be relatively unaffected. If you feel that you are 'in limbo', not knowing what will happen to you and your research project, and your named supervisor is not clear about this, then raise your concerns with someone else involved in the research project part of the curriculum. Ultimately your institution has a responsibility towards the students and you should be provided with an opportunity for a good research project, even if it is not as originally envisaged.

From time-to-time, a student and their supervisor may have a clash of personalities that leads to a poor working relationship. This is no different from any other pair of colleagues failing to get along, and there is no 'one size fits all' universal solution. It is a fact of life that we cannot expect everyone to see things as we do, or have the same attitude to work and working relationships. When there is conflict between a student and a supervisor, this usually arises because of a mismatch of expectations. If your institution is one where supervisors make a decision to offer projects, then your supervisor clearly is motivated to take a student for a research project. In contrast, in an institution where it is compulsory for the supervisor to offer a project, he or she may see the project student rather differently. As a professional, the supervisor should provide the student with the necessary support and guidance, regardless of how the situation arose, and the vast majority of supervisors will do this. Good supervisors will recognise which students are lacking in confidence or ability and adjust their supervisory style to account for this. Sometimes, however, a student and a supervisor can have big misunderstandings. Consider the following pairs of statements:

- **Student:** All I said was 'Has there been anything published recently in this area?'
- **Supervisor A:** 'He expects me to do his literature search for him!'
- **Supervisor B:** 'I had to explain that it was his responsibility to keep abreast of the literature.'

- **Student:** 'I spent 3 days doing exactly what she told me and I got no results at all.'
- **Supervisor A:** 'I gave her a simple task, and she wasted 3 days getting NO results, and she never thought to come and tell me the experiment wasn't working.'
- **Supervisor B:** 'She spent 3 days struggling with the practical work. What a shame she never thought to let me know it wasn't working. At least she has a thorough understanding of the equipment now.'

- **Student:** 'I thought it would be worthwhile asking Dr Smith to have a look at my slides, since he gave us the lectures in the first year, and when he found out, my supervisor went ballistic.'
- **Supervisor A:** 'Instead of discussing his slides with me, the idiot took his slides to Dr Smith, who knows nothing about the topic, and gave completely the wrong interpretation of the data, and had the audacity to suggest (in

front of the head of department) that I should not be supervising a project in this area.'

- **Supervisor B:** 'He should have discussed his findings with me first, since Dr Smith isn't involved in his project, but we talked about this and he won't repeat that mistake.'

- **Student:** 'I sent her a draft of the first section of my dissertation and it took her 3 weeks to give feedback.'
- **Supervisor A:** 'She sent me something at the beginning of the month that fell off my radar, and instead of speaking to me she went to the module leader and said I wasn't giving feedback within the time frame laid down in the regulations!'
- **Supervisor B:** 'I had to explain to her that I am very busy just at the moment and that, if I overlook an e-mail, she should feel free to remind me, or resend.'

It is obvious that each trio of statements indicates that the student and supervisor A are not working in harmony! Supervisor B has a different (and preferable) attitude and outlook to Supervisor A. In the examples shown above, any blame for the situation involving Supervisor A could be divided between student and supervisor. The take-home point from this is that supervisors are not angels and sometimes have unreasonable expectations. As the student, you also have a responsibility towards building a good working relationship, and should acknowledge that your supervisor is only human and may misjudge matters from time to time. The key to building and maintaining a working relationship is good communication, which means that you give your supervisor regular updates on your progress and are never reluctant to bring difficulties to his or her attention – together with any suggestions you may have to overcome these. In those rare situations where there is a real breakdown in the relationship between the student and the supervisor, then a third party can be brought in to mediate and bring an understanding of what each party will do to ensure that the project gets back on track. This person may be your mentor, course leader or head of department. It is rare for students to invoke formal complaints about their supervisors (though the procedures will exist for this to take place) and wherever possible, it is best to use the informal procedures to set matters straight so that you can concentrate on the really important matter – which is your research project and dissertation.

Problems relating to yourself

The problems students face during the times they are working on their research projects are often the same as during any other part of their studies, including – but not limited to – health (theirs or that of a family member or close friend), money or personal relationships. What each person needs to ask themselves is whether their personal problem affects their ability to carry out their project to the expected high standard. In some cases the issue is irrelevant – a student that needs to deliver pizzas a couple of evenings a week to help pay the rent is not likely to find that it has a major impact on their work. The student who is facing eviction for non-payment of rent is in a different situation. Someone with a chronic medical condition that is stable and well controlled may feel that it has no bearing on their work or project: a student who has a hospital admission as a result of that condition (sickle cell crisis, severe exacerbation of asthma) may see things differently.

Health problems

When any student has a health problem affecting their work, they owe it to themselves to seek out appropriate support. As someone planning a career in medicine or healthcare, you should appreciate the need to take care of your own well-being. This includes mental health issues; people working in health-related professions are just as likely to have problems related to mental health as anyone else. If you are not registered with a GP then the Student Health Centre (or equivalent) at your institution should be your first port of call. Do keep a note of medical appointments or consultations so that you are able to demonstrate when your health problems began, should you be in the position of wanting to ask for an extension to your project. If you require time away from your studies for medical reasons, you will need a note from a healthcare provider to justify this. If your medical problem is of a highly personal nature or you want the details to be confidential, you can specify this, so that (for example) only your supervisor, course convenor and chair of the exam board might know why you have requested an extension to your project.

Family illness or bereavement

Sometimes the health problem is not your own, but relates to a family member, and it may be that you are spending a lot of time in supporting your family in practical ways. Bereavement can happen at any time, and nobody can know in advance how they will be affected by the death of someone close. Naturally, many people feel that their place is with their family when things are tough. When this is the case, a student can feel very torn about their obligations. There may be cultural differences in what is expected of individuals at times of family crises, so that students facing apparently similar problems may feel a different sense of obligation. For everyone, it is sometimes difficult to see things objectively when caught up in stressful (and distressing) situations, and it can help enormously to have support from others who can help you to keep a proper perspective. In addition to your friends, speak to your supervisor so that he or she is aware of the difficulties you are facing. If you do not feel comfortable talking to your supervisor, find another member of staff such as your mentor or personal tutor, who you feel you can talk to freely and ask their advice about how to balance work and family responsibilities.

Financial problems

What constitutes a significant financial problem may vary from one person to another, because we all have a different threshold of what level of debt will keep us awake at night. If you are seriously concerned about your finances, make an appointment with the Student Welfare Office for some clear advice. They have the knowledge and expertise to help. If you have significant financial problems these are unlikely to have arisen overnight, and Welfare Officers can help you to develop a strategy to move into a better financial position. A sudden financial crisis can arise out of the blue, such as finding that you are the victim of stolen identity, your bank cards cease to work and someone has run up a huge debt on your account. In this kind of situation, you will most likely be in communication with your bank and possibly the police, but such situations often take considerable time to be resolved. Meanwhile, you may not have cash for the basics of daily living. You may have family or friends who can help in these circumstances and your Student Welfare Office may be able to advise you on other potential sources of financial support, or even provide a hardship loan in extreme circumstances.

Personal or relationship issues

Relationship difficulties are part of life and may be particularly common in young adulthood. If you are going through a difficult time it is to be hoped that your friends and family will provide the necessary support and your personal problems will not affect your work. If the break-up of a long-standing relationship or other personal problem is seriously affecting how you are functioning, then consider making an appointment with the student counselling service, or other counselling service via your GP. These services are confidential and non-judgemental and should help you to work through the pain and move forward.

Who needs to know when a student has problems?

If you are facing personal problems and are unsure about whether you should disclose them to your supervisor or discuss them with anyone else, remember that supervisors can only be supportive if they know what is happening. If a student is always late, miserable, often absent and unreliable, the supervisor may just get very annoyed. If the supervisor knows there is an underlying major problem, he or she can point the way to external support services and discuss with the student how to address the problem in the best way. Put yourself in the position of the supervisor: would you rather know that your student

- had a significant medical condition?
- was in the middle of a major financial crisis?
- was spending every weekend visiting a parent with a terminal illness?
- had just broken up with a long-standing partner?
- had been sharing a house with another student who had committed suicide?
- was facing a criminal prosecution?

Anything from the list above is likely to have consequences on how the student performs and therefore, arguably, should be disclosed. Good supervisors do not need or want to know the details of the private lives of their students (nor of any other colleagues, for that matter) but where these affect performance, they are relevant. How easy or difficult it is to speak to your supervisor will depend on how well you know him or her and how approachable he or she is. If it is something you cannot face up to, then speak to another staff member that you do feel comfortable with, in the first instance, and he or she should be able to help you find the best way forward in communicating with your supervisor. The members of academic staff are not usually in a position to provide specialist advice, but they should be able to point the way to any relevant institutional sources of support that can help you. Remember that the support services of your institution (Welfare Office, Health Centre, Counselling Service, Chaplaincy, etc.) are there specifically to provide help when needed. Use them.

Sometimes health or personal problems mean that a student cannot complete their project in the allocated time, or the amount of work written up or presented is less than expected. Where this is likely to be the case, the sooner it is known the easier it is to find a solution that is fair to the student while maintaining academic standards. It is difficult to conceive of solutions to all possible eventualities, although an extension is an obvious solution to some. The staff with responsibilities for the research project part of the curriculum will have a responsibility to find the best solution in any set of unforeseen circumstances, and of course they will take your views into consideration. In almost all cases a satisfactory solution is worked out. Occasionally, a student may feel that the decision made is not the one they wanted. The student might feel that they should be allowed to continue writing up their project in parallel with returning to the next stage of the curriculum. Instead they are given a shorter extension and perhaps asked to submit their dissertation at the end of a vacation, at a stage when they feel it would benefit from more work. Sometimes the student will think that he or she needs only a short time to complete their work, but the supervisor recommends a longer extension, which brings less pressure. In such situations, it is worth remembering that the staff are really working with your best interests at heart, have probably spent considerable time looking at different options and seeking institutional approval for the proposed course of action. They have the benefit of experience and the student may come to realise this, albeit at a later stage.

Monitoring, assessment and procedural issues

Very occasionally there may be problems of a procedural nature. Examples might be that forms relating to your project are not submitted on time or some information is lacking. In many cases this is of no consequence and the students will be unaware that things were not done according to the letter of the law. Where you may be concerned about adherence to procedures is in the matter of your assessment. If you feel that any matter relating to your research project has been improperly conducted, you will need to check the relevant regulations carefully to see if this was indeed the case. As a general rule, students are not allowed to challenge the academic judgement of their assessors, but can seek redress if procedures did not comply with the regulations. If you are in this situation and decide to appeal against the outcome of your assessment, you must be reasonably sure that whatever was wrong in your assessment was in clear breach of the regulations and substantially affected the outcome of your assessment. Such occasions are unusual and your supervisor may be unfamiliar with the relevant regulations; you may need to check with senior administrative staff about what you need to do to challenge the grading of your project. Such procedures are not usually quick. If your challenge is upheld, you may find yourself being reassessed some considerable time after completing your project, so you should be certain of your grounds before embarking on any challenge to the assessment of your research project.

SUMMARY

Expect the unexpected. Problems can arise even in the best-planned projects. Be alert to practical difficulties relating to your project and take steps at an early stage to ameliorate these, particularly if they are holding up essential progress. If one part of your project is 'on hold', ensure that you use the time to make progress with others.

Be proactive in sorting out the practical problems wherever possible, and do not expect others to do this for you.

Difficulties can arise if a supervisor is unexpectedly unable to fulfil their obligations to the student. Your institution has an obligation to support each student and alternative supervision may be put in place, though this may necessitate modification to your project.

Supervisors are not angels. Problems between students and supervisors usually arise because of a mismatch of expectations and/or poor communication. Keep your supervisor updated on what you are doing and meet up regularly. If there are real difficulties in your working relationship, seek the advice of someone such as your mentor or the course leader.

Where a student has personal problems that affect their ability to perform to their best, this should be disclosed. The members of academic staff should be able to point you in the direction of the institutional sources of support. Your college or university will have a range of student support services. Use them.

Where you believe that proper procedure has not been followed with regard to your project and that you have been disadvantaged by that, you will have the right to appeal, for example, against the mark you have been awarded. Check the relevant institutional regulations very carefully before submitting an appeal, and be certain of your case.

THE LAST WORD

Your research project is likely to be one of the things you remember best from your time as a student. Unlike most of your formal teaching, such as 'systems' modules, it will give you the opportunity to work with a considerable degree of independence. It will make demands on you that you never envisaged. At times, it will drive you crackers. At the end of it, however, if you have fully engaged with your project and given it your total commitment, you will emerge not only with a great dissertation but with a much enhanced understanding of how research 'works' and, I hope, a strong desire to do more. Make the most of it. Go for it, and enjoy it.

Index

How to do your Research Project: A Guide for Students in Medicine and the Health Sciences,
First Edition. Caroline Beardsmore.
© 2013 John Wiley & Sons, Ltd. Published 2013 by John Wiley & Sons, Ltd.